PRIORITY SETTING:
The Health Care Debate

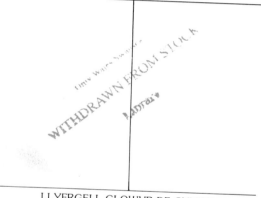

PRIORITY SETTING: The Health Care Debate

Edited by

Joanna Coast

Jenny Donovan

and

Stephen Frankel

University of Bristol, UK

JOHN WILEY & SONS

Chichester · New York · Brisbane · Toronto · Singapore

Other Wiley Editorial Offices

John Wiley & Sons, Inc., 605 Third Avenue,
New York, NY 10158-0012, USA

Jacaranda Wiley Ltd, 33 Park Road, Milton,
Queensland 4064, Australia

John Wiley & Sons (Canada) Ltd, 22 Worcester Road,
Rexdale, Ontario M9W 1L1, Canada

John Wiley & Sons (Asia) Pte Ltd, 2 Clementi Loop #02-01,
Jin Xing Distripark, Singapore 0512

Library of Congress Cataloging-in-Publication Data

Priority setting : the health care debate / edited by Joanna
    Coast, Jenny Donovan, and Stephen Frankel.
        p.   cm.
    Includes bibliographical references and index.
    ISBN 0-471-96102-7 (hardcover)
    1. Medical policy.   2. Health care rationing.   3. Right to health
    care.   4. Medical policy—Great Britain—Citizen participation.
    I. Coast, Joanna.   II. Donovan, Jenny, *1960–* .   III. Frankel,
    Stephen.
    RA393.P763   1996
    362.1—dc20   95–42635
                                                                  CIP

British Library Cataloguing in Publication Data

A catalogue record for this book is available from the British Library

ISBN 0-471-96102-7

Typeset in 11/13pt Palatino by Mackreth Media Services, Hemel Hempstead, Herts
Printed and bound in Great Britain by Biddles Ltd, Guildford and King's Lynn
This book is printed on acid-free paper responsibly manufactured from sustainable forestation,
for which at least two trees are planted for each one used for paper production.

Contents

Contributors

Gwyn Bevan
Joanna Coast
Jenny Donovan
Stephen Frankel
Ian Harvey
Ben Toth

Department of Social Medicine, University of Bristol, Canynge Hall, Whiteladies Road, Bristol BS8 2PR, UK

0117 928 7279.

Preface

This book starts from the premise that priority setting is surrounded by conflict and confusion, fuelled by rhetoric. The aspiration of satisfying a population's potential demand for health care is no longer entertained seriously. During the postwar years the combination of economic growth and significant advances in preventive and curative medicine supported a somewhat uncritical enhancement of the volume of care. Areas of expansion were guided to a significant extent by the preferences of clinicians, while public policy was designed largely to facilitate this clinician-led expansion. Over the past two decades three strands have combined to undermine this consensus.

First the slowing, and in some cases reversal, of economic growth has resulted in general constraints upon public expenditure. The choices in health care therefore concern areas of exclusion as well as the more comfortable choices between options for expansion.

Second, the critique of medicine informed by epidemiologists, social scientists, economists, historians and jurists has led to a more questioning environment for health policy. The assumption that more health care is necessarily preferable no longer holds. The assertions of clinicians must now in general be supported by more formal evidence.

Third, widespread prosperity has brought with it greater expectations amongst consumers that their preferences for goods and services should be satisfied. Organisations purporting to represent such consumer views have become active in many areas, including health care.

These various strands have come together in a number of propositions that are no longer in serious contention in debates concerning health policy. These propositions can be summarised as follows: resources are finite; the potential demand for health care is infinite; not all forms of health care are equally effective, indeed some are positively harmful; means of delivery of health care may not be efficient; the provision of health care should reflect the preferences of the population.

These propositions lead to a conclusion which is simple to state: the balance of care should be adjusted to ensure that health care expenditure is efficiently devoted to the provision of those interventions which are effective and desired by the population. While this unexceptionable aspiration is clear, the means for acting upon it, particularly in any local context, are exceedingly unclear. Indeed many individuals who through their positions have accepted implicit responsibility for this task are quite unsure as to how they might discharge it.

There is of course no simple recipe for achieving what ultimately implies the resolution of the conflicting wishes of individuals, for one person's rational choice may require the denial of another's. Nevertheless the current level of uncertainty as to how to move, however hesitantly, towards this goal seems so great that some outline of the policy options may have value in assisting those bodies and individuals concerned with local policy.

The analysis presented here is therefore offered as a guide to policy and action. However, policy and action cannot succeed in this extraordinarily complex area without an adequate understanding of the conflicting and sometimes confusing issues involved. For this reason the book is divided into five parts, providing a critical review of the various disciplinary contributions that can be brought to bear upon the major issues.

Part One *The context* provides the essential contextual information required for an understanding of the debate about rationing and priority setting in health care.

Chapter One sets the scene, raising and discussing the conflicts and confusion inherent in priority setting. Themes developed in this chapter recur throughout the book, particularly the apparent complexity arising from the rhetoric associated with conflicts between such major issues as implicit and explicit rationing, technical or pluralistic bargaining methods for determining priorities, equity and efficiency as bases for priority setting, and public participation and medical paternalism as they impinge on priority-setting exercises.

Part Two *From implicit to explicit rationing: two steps forward and one step back* provides further context for the debate by focusing first on empirical examples of priority setting and then considering the philosophical basis for such exercises.

Chapters Two and Three examine two steps forward in the debate. The examples, from Oregon in the USA and New Zealand, show how priority setting has, in practice, moved on from theory to practice. They also, of course, provide valuable information for future attempts to set priorities. The two empirical examples have been chosen because, although both provide examples of explicit priority setting, they are based in the very different traditions of technical priority setting (Oregon) and pluralistic bargaining (New Zealand). By far the most ambitious and most discussed of all the priority-setting attempts has been that of the US state of Oregon. Here the aim was to set priorities across all health care interventions using technical methodologies. In contrast, New Zealand's attempt to define Core Services has been largely overlooked by the international academic community. Although the two chapters illuminate many differences between these two attempts to set priorities, the need to compromise at several different levels is common to both.

Chapter Four represents a "step back" in that it describes vital background information concerning the ethical basis of priority-setting exercises. The chapter describes the tensions between the various philosophical perspectives underlying the ethical positions from which the priority-setting debate can be conducted. Deontology, consequentialism and equity are each discussed in relation to the health policy debate. It is clear that this rather stereotypical group of models does not correspond in any easy one-to-one fashion with the views and problems of the priority-setting arena. Inevitably, however, each of these philosophical perspectives will impinge upon the choice between implicit and explicit priority setting, the preferred means of explicit priority setting and also the conflicts between equity and efficiency, and between paternalism and lay participation.

Part Three *Technical priority setting and the equity–efficiency conflict* reviews and appraises two of the major methods of priority setting: efficiency and equity. In Chapter Five, the economic contribution to priority setting is described and analysed. The discussion centres on two methods for priority setting which have their ethical basis in utilitarianism, and which aim to maximise the benefit from the limited funding available for health care. These two methods are cost–utility analysis (with outcome measured in terms of QALYs, or quality-adjusted life-years) and programme budgeting and marginal analysis. Chapter Six is similar to Chapter Five, except that it concentrates upon the technical priority-setting models which have their ethical basis in equity, rather than efficiency, principles. The following bases for setting priorities are discussed: equal access for equal need; equal access for equal age. What is clear from these two chapters is that technical models tend to be based on one principle and do not generally involve trading off one objective against another.

Part Four *Pluralistic bargaining and public participation* outlines the major issues and conflicts arising from the desire to incorporate a lay perspective into priority-setting exercises, set within an historical context. In Chapter Seven, an historical analysis of health care in the UK indicates that lay involvement was gradually and systematically eroded until the late 1980s. Chapter Eight details the changes in government policy since that date. It also describes many crucial yet neglected issues associated with public participation in priority setting, focusing particularly on whether obtaining a representative view of the public is an illusion, and the degree to which there is real commitment to it from government and local health authorities.

Part Five *A way forward* presents a practical approach to setting priorities using current evidence. Chapter Nine provides a clarification of the issues contained in the book. In particular, it advocates an acceptance of the inevitable conflicts inherent in rationing and priority setting, while at the same time offering an approach for the present and future. This is the model of health care requirements, which aims explicitly to combine the best of the traditions of pluralistic bargaining and technical bargaining, and to draw together the various threads in priority setting.

Joanna Coast
Jenny Donovan
Stephen Frankel

Acknowledgements

We would like to acknowledge the help of the following in commenting on earlier drafts of chapters of the book: Richard Smith, Stephen Clarke, Kieran Morgan, Ken Buckingham, Max Bachman, Tim Peters, Max Kammerling, Steve Sturdy.

PART ONE

The Context

CHAPTER ONE

JOANNA COAST AND JENNY DONOVAN

Conflict, Complexity and Confusion: The Context for Priority Setting

Without a bowel transplant from birth a small child will probably die. The total cost of treatment, including seven new organs, is estimated at around £1 million.[1] Should she be treated?

A young girl has leukaemia and has received treatment that has been ineffective. Further treatment is estimated to provide a chance of survival of between 2 and 20%.[2] Should she be treated?

One hospital has had, for ten years, a policy that smokers should not receive coronary artery bypass grafting.[1] When this policy becomes public, debate ensues as to whether this is the edge of the slippery slope[3-5] or a sensible policy based on the effectiveness of treatment in different groups of patients?[6,7]

These recent examples taken from the UK illustrate some of the complexities associated with priority setting in health care. The examples do not reflect a sustained and public debate about the rationing of health care. Rather they are the bubblings of a volcano which seems constantly on the verge of eruption yet inexplicably subsides following each small explosion.

This chapter examines these complexities, aiming to expose the tensions implicit in different positions. Only with clarity of thought

Priority Setting: The Health Care Debate.
Edited by J. Coast, J. Donovan and S. Frankel.   © 1996 John Wiley & Sons Ltd.

and acknowledgement of the different values which may quite legitimately be held, will the aim of explicit priority setting in health care be advanced. To date there has been little acceptance of the validity of opposing views in this area, nor has there been a clear overview of these different positions and how they relate to one another. Figure 1.1 shows the structure of this whole area in the form of a decision tree relating to the various conflicts and tensions between alternative positions. Proponents of different approaches have tended to focus on only one branch of this tree, in some cases to such an extent that their main interest has appeared to be in "selling" their own priority setting "branch" (for example, see Mooney et al,[8] Hunter[9]). This tendency has contributed to the apparent complexity.

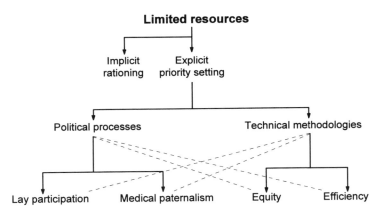

Figure 1.1   A structure for priority setting

The chapter begins with a discussion of the terminology of rationing, and questions whether there is, and will be, rationing of health care: this question is dismissed relatively easily, and the real question of whether rationing should become explicit or should remain implicit is then examined. If the answer to this question is that rationing should be made more explicit, there are major sources of both confusion and conflict which must be addressed and which are discussed in detail. There is a question of whether rationing should have a technical basis, or should be based on the political process. Each of these alternatives exposes a further conflict: in the case of technical rationing the conflict between equity and efficiency as principles upon which to base priority setting is revealed; in the case of rationing via the political process it is the question of the extent to which decisions should be based on medical or lay opinion. The dashed lines on Figure 1.1, however, show that both conflicts exist for both types of rationing, although they are less clear. These themes will not only be discussed in detail here, but will, to a greater or lesser extent, recur throughout the remaining chapters of the book.

TO RATION OR NOT TO RATION: IS THAT THE QUESTION?

Rationing is an emotive term, evoking for many memories of wartime, coupons, and a lack of basic necessities. For those of us fortunate enough to be spared such memories and accustomed throughout our lives to a consumer society the idea of "rationing" may be equally worrying. After all, don't we all have a right to health care through the NHS?

Application of the terminology of "rationing" to health care for many people implies severe cuts in provision. The rationing of health care does not, however, (at least for those of us living in the developed world) equate to an immediate and harsh austerity. It is merely a statement that not every possible action to improve health could be undertaken, and so decisions must be made about how to allocate the resources available for health care. As Alberti and Tudor Hart state, health care rationing refers to "any planning, resource allocation or pruning of ineffective or unproved processes".[10] Health care thus compares to other areas of life: there is no talk of the rationing of defence or education, yet society is aware that the funds for these activities are not unlimited. Although the terminology of "rationing" has not been used, rationing does indeed take place. Decisions are made about how to allocate the limited resources available, just as they are for health care. Rationing is thus merely another term for stating that we must decide how to allocate our limited resources.

In a free market, decisions about how to allocate health care resources would not arise. It is because of the lack of a market system that there is the need for society to make rationing-type decisions, that is, there is the need to make decisions about how to allocate health care resources. If health care was purchased on the same basis as food, another basic necessity for life, no discussion about priorities would be required (although obviously individuals would be required to determine their own priorities for expenditure). Individuals would buy a procedure to remove an ingrowing toe-nail on much the same basis as they buy a joint of beef or a tofu meal. They would set their own priorities. For very many good (and obvious) reasons, societies generally choose not to use this system of allocation for health care. Among others, these reasons include our uncertainty about both the timing and extent of our health care needs which make it difficult to plan for purchasing health care; the great expense associated with purchasing many health care procedures; and the fact that patients do not usually know what services they need to receive. Thus in all nations, at the very least, health care insurance is available, and in the majority of societies there is also government intervention. Most of us would not choose a system whereby health care was purchased directly because, among other reasons, we would not like the allocation that such a system would provide – with the rich able to purchase health care, and the poor unable to do so. Just because we choose not to have this form of allocation, however, does not mean that we can absolve ourselves from having to make any choices at all. Unfortunately, rejecting the direct purchase of health care is not the same as ensuring unlimited provision for all.

Both rationing as described above, and the related notion of resource scarcity, are inexorably linked with priority setting in health care. There would be no need to set priorities if the resources existed to do everything desirable. All care which was needed and/or demanded would be provided to all patients. Health care is not available in unlimited supply, however, and so there is a need to decide who receives what share of the available health care supply. This is the "rationing" of health care.

It has often been stated that there is no necessity to ration the delivery of health care services.[11-13] Those who state that rationing is unnecessary usually put forward some alternative method by which health care can be increased without rationing. In the US context this may be increased public financial input,[11] or the reduction of waste and the improvement of the present health care system.[12-14] In the

UK it is often stated that there would be no requirement for rationing if the resources allocated to health care were increased in line with other developed nations.[15]

There is, as evidenced by these arguments, a basic confusion between different proponents about the terminology of rationing. For example, even if resources in the UK were increased in line with other countries, there would still be the need to make decisions about the allocation of resources to different health care procedures, in other words, to ration. Health care rationing as defined here and elsewhere is the failure to provide all beneficial care to all people.[16] There is already a failure to provide all such care,[17,18] with implicit and unacknowledged rationing occurring in all health systems (some examples are given later in this chapter).

There is the expectation that the extent of rationing may need to increase as a result of the increasing capabilities of modern medicine, an ageing population and rising expectations.[19] This prospect has heightened national and international interest in, and acceptance of, health care rationing. The need to ration health care has now been formally acknowledged in a number of countries (for example The Netherlands,[20] New Zealand[21]) and there is an international interest in the explicit setting of priorities. In the UK implicit acceptance of priority setting in health care has been provided recently by both doctors[22] and Secretaries of State for Health.[23] In the USA high health care costs (12.3% of GNP in 1992[24]), combined with incomplete coverage of the population have led to a greater debate about the need for rationing than in many other countries. Although there are those who maintain that there is no need to ration, many hold views like those of Daniel Callahan, who feels that there will not be the ability to pay for increasing amounts of health care in the future, nor for endlessly emerging life-extending technologies, particularly among the ageing population.[25,26]

The *extent* to which health care provision needs to be limited *is* however a question for debate. Knowledge about the effectiveness of different procedures, although improving, is still relatively poor and there are commentators who feel that rationing would not be required if effective interventions only were pursued.[27] It might also be, however, that even a system which only provided "effective" health care would need to ration care.

It should be apparent from both the commentary in this section and the size of this book, that there is agreement amongst the authors that rationing will occur – that is, that there is, and will continue to be, a failure to provide all beneficial care to all people. Acceptance of this fact does not, however, equate to the expectation that the "infinite demand" which has in the past been attributed to health care will suddenly require extreme cut-backs in the care that is already provided.[27] Rather, it is a matter of questioning how decisions about the allocation of care should be made. Whether or not there should be rationing is not, in fact, the important question for two main reasons. First, the need for health care rationing has been accepted across most of the developed world. Second, and more importantly, "to ration or not to ration" is a misrepresentation of the real question, which concerns whether rationing should be implicit or explicit.

WHAT'S IN A NAME? EXPLICIT VERSUS IMPLICIT RATIONING

As there has been growing acceptance of rationing in health care, interest in *explicit* priority setting has increased among academics, health care professionals and politicians. The desire for explicit priority setting has resulted from the increasing acceptance across many different communities and nations that not all health care can be provided for all individuals, in conjunction with a realisation that decisions are not necessarily made in the "best" ways possible at present.

What is the distinction to be made between implicit and explicit rationing? Implicit rationing is often mistakenly equated with an absence of rationing, whilst explicit rationing is assumed to mean the introduction of a policy to ration health care. Implicit rationing is, however, the unacknowledged limitation of care, inevitably occurring where there is no explicit rationing: the volcanic eruptions are the few instances in which implicit rationing becomes an explicit statement that treatment will not be provided. Implicit is defined as "implied though not plainly expressed"[28] or "not explicit" where explicit is defined as "precisely and clearly expressed".[29] In terms of rationing this means that where neither the decisions themselves, nor the bases for those decisions, are clearly expressed, rationing is implicit.

There are valid reasons why a policy of implicit rationing might be preferred to a policy of explicit rationing – not least the comfort of Ministers! This section provides a discussion of the implicit rationing systems which currently exist, as well as examining the views of those whose aim is to encourage explicit priority setting. Before entering this discussion, however, it is important to make the point that explicit rationing is unlikely ever to replace implicit rationing entirely: wholly implicit and wholly explicit rationing are two ends of a continuum. It is the extent to which a society wishes to move along this continuum that is important.

IMPLICIT RATIONING

There are many ways of allocating health care resources, within two organisational extremes. First, allocation of scarce resources in health care may take place through the market system, with allocation by price according to the interaction of demand and supply. Second, allocation of resources may take place through a centrally funded system according to any one or more criteria which may be either explicitly stated or implicit. Within either allocation system clinicians will influence the rationing process. Where allocation takes place through a centrally funded system, rationing may be implicit in that it is not acknowledged and takes place according to no particular criteria, or it may be explicit.

Methods of distributing health care are generally implicit at present, with no sense among the public that rationing is occurring and no specific statements about the care which will or will not be provided. In different cultural settings the perception of what constitutes implicit rationing and what is explicit may be very different. This fact is illustrated in the discussions below of implicit rationing in the two organisational extremes of the USA and the UK. Although examples of implicit rationing are taken only from these two countries, such examples could equally have come from accounts of any health care system.

In the USA the general perception has been that there is no rationing of health care. Here, the centrally funded Medicaid system is intended to provide care for the poorest in society – those below the federal poverty line. There is an upper limit on the resources available, however, and insufficient funds are available for all those below the poverty line to receive care. In the USA this has not been seen as a policy of rationing, perhaps because the state absolves itself of responsibility for those not covered by Medicaid. These individuals are responsible for providing their own health care and it is, perhaps, assumed that those who do not have insurance have chosen to be uninsured – rather than that their care is being rationed in any way.

There is the perception in the UK, however, that ". . .the United States already rations health care somewhat brutally. . ." (Klein,[30] p.144), by failing to provide medical care for many of those below the poverty line who are unable to purchase their own medical insurance. The implicit priority upheld by the Medicaid system is that health care resources should be allocated according to inability to pay, and the Medicaid programme has been described as making:

> a list of poor people, with those who are poorest at the top. Depending on how much money is available for Medicaid, states draw a line partway down the list of people. People above the line are eligible for Medicaid; those below the line are not. Medicaid then provides virtually unlimited health care to people above the line, but nothing to people below the line. There is no effort to discriminate between health services that are essential and effective and those of marginal or unknown value. (Rooks,[31] p.43)

The extent of health care rationing through this system is relatively large: the level of inability to pay required to be eligible for Medicaid is set separately from state to state, and has tended to be redefined downwards since Medicaid was introduced in 1965. The proportion of poor people covered by Medicaid has declined from a high of about 65% to less than 40% at present.[32] In one state, Alabama, the income threshold for eligibility is as low as 14% of the federal poverty level.[33] Approximately 35 million (17.5% of those aged under 65) individuals in the USA have no health insurance and do not receive Medicare or Medicaid.[34]

In the UK nobody is completely excluded from state health services. There is still, however, extensive implicit rationing of health care. This is in part a reflection of the lower expenditure on health care in the UK compared with many other similarly developed nations. The 6% of national income spent on health care in the UK[35] is less than half that spent in the USA, and considerably less than in most other European countries.[36] Some academics considering the question of explicit priority setting in the UK National Health Service have concluded that such a process would only be seen to be "fair" when the UK spends as much on health care as the rest of the European Community.[15]

In the UK, there may be little or no impression among the public that rationing of health care takes place on a daily basis (other than for elective surgery through the waiting list) but this is certainly the perception among commentators from other systems of health care provision. For example:

> Per capita spending on health care, about one-third in Britain of that in the United States, requires a degree of rationing there far beyond any that is conceivable here [United States]. (Aaron and Schwartz,[35] p.420)

> . . .the British experience with rationing, particularly stark because of its severity. . . (Aaron and Schwartz,[35] p.422)

> Rationing in Great Britain has been implicit. . . It is a silent conspiracy between a dense, obscurating bureaucracy, intentionally avoiding written policy for macroallocation (rationing), and a publicly unaccountable medical profession privately managing microallocation so as to conceal life and death decisions from patients. (Crawshaw,[37] p.663)

In the UK health care system, which is centrally funded and limited on the supply-side, rationing must be effected by some means other than price. There is considerable evidence that rationing in the UK is at present implicit;[18,38] for example, the fact that the elderly have been much less likely to receive renal dialysis in the UK than in the

USA has not occurred as the result of an official policy of denying care, but as a result of a limited number of machines and staff to run them,[39] and referral practices which acknowledge this fact. Rationing in the UK is carried out by physicians who are aware of budgetary limits, but who ration care by telling the patient that they are unable to do anything to help them, rather than explicitly stating that the resources are not available for treatment.[18,30,40–42] Instead the denial of care is made to seem optimal or routine, with the assertion that the treatment given is medically optimal and that patients denied care or given alternative forms of care for financial reasons do not suffer a loss of health as a result.[18,43] Aaron and Schwarz state that this "enables doctors to avoid the painful realisation that they are doing less than the best for the patient"(Aaron and Schwarz,[18] p.101). As many patients may be unaware that their care is being rationed, it may be that physicians in the UK accept that the utility of both their patients and themselves would be reduced by an admission that treatment was not forthcoming because of a lack of resources.

Much rationing takes place at the point of access to the health care system. The role of the General Practitioner (GP) in the UK is one of gatekeeper to the system: in particular the GP is able to control access to specialist services. The wide variations in GP referral patterns that exist[44,45] may reflect different referral criteria and/or the different attitudes of GPs to their role in rationing health care.

As rationing is not explicit, there is no real awareness of the principles being used to ration health care, or, in other words, to set priorities. In the case of kidney dialysis, for example, it is not evident whether the implicit priority upon which the past denial of dialysis to the elderly has been based, is:

1. The young should be given priority over the old.
2. Those obtaining greater medical benefit should be given priority over those obtaining lesser medical benefit.
3. Those with greater ability to cope with dialysis should be given priority over those less able to cope with dialysis.
4. Those with a greater life expectancy should be given priority over those with a shorter life expectancy.
5. Some combination of the above.
6. Some other priority base.

Klein has stated that health care in the UK has been rationed according to medically defined need,[30] but it has also been asserted that, in practice, the NHS implicitly prioritises against the old, the working class and women.[43] It is almost certainly the case that different priorities are used in different areas, and also that doctors have varying levels of efficiency in applying their own priorities. Studies of medical practice variations have frequently demonstrated the existence of variation at every level of aggregation. It is likely that the application of different priorities contributes to this variation in treatment rates by location.

In the UK, there has been little central direction regarding the setting of priorities but, with the introduction of the health service reforms, it has become inevitable that explicit priorities are at least considered as an option by many health authorities. The discussion of the issues involved in setting priorities is only of a preliminary nature, however. There are many issues hidden behind the assumptions that these activities should, and can, become part of the activity of purchasing authorities, particularly when making some services a priority involves denoting other services of low priority. It remains to be seen whether political support will be forthcoming for making rationing more visible.

SHOULD RATIONING BE MORE EXPLICIT?

What is meant by explicit rationing? In its most narrow sense, it could refer to the making of lists of conditions that will not be treated. It is in this sense that Redmayne et al refer to explicit rationing.[46] Here, however, the meaning of explicit rationing is somewhat broader. Explicit rationing is concerned with making clear the decisions that have been made about resource allocation *and* the basis upon which these decisions have been made. This means that explicit rationing may encompass both "technical" methods, such as those often associated with economists, and also the methods of political bargaining.

Where rationing is explicit it may also be known as priority setting and this term will be used here to denote the use of explicit systems for the distribution of scarce health care resources. Although implicit priorities are at present incorporated into most systems, implicit rationing will not be included in the definition of priority setting as used in this document. Implicit rationing is not part of the process of setting priorities, although it will inevitably affect the final distribution of resources.

In the UK the reorganisation of the health service on the basis of an internal market has made those both within and outside the health services more aware of the choice to be made between implicit rationing and explicit priority setting. The split between purchasing and providing roles means that, to some extent, the responsibility for rationing has passed to purchasers and away from hospital consultants. The purchasers of health care, including both health authorities and GP fundholders, are now responsible for "ensuring that the health needs of the population for which they are responsible are met" (Department of Health,[47] p.14). They must decide what to buy and what not to buy, and thus they have a role at the planning level in making decisions about rationing and the setting of priorities.

In the present political climate, in which rights are emphasised through such publications as the Patient's Charter,[48] there is a case for making choices more explicit, and this opportunity is welcomed by many. Alan Maynard declares that "It is time that the issue of rationing was approached logically and explicitly and that priorities were set within the framework of cost-effectiveness" (Maynard,[49] p.19). The editor of the *British Medical Journal*, Richard Smith, has stated that "Although it is tempting to leave the decisions to be fudged by kindly professionals, I believe that we should follow the Oregonians into the sunlight" (Smith,[42] p.1562). There are, however, also opponents to those wishing priorities to be set explicitly. Sir Raymond Hoffenberg maintains the traditional view that "If services are to be limited, I would rather see it done implicitly – unstated, unwritten, unacknowledged – in the curious and not inhumane way in which such matters are managed in the United Kingdom" (quoted in Smith,[42] p.1562).

Although there is a choice to be made about whether priorities in the NHS should continue to be implicit or should be set explicitly, many believe that the new purchasing process in the NHS will lead to explicit rationing.[50] Certainly there has been increased interest in the issues surrounding priority setting in recent years.[8,9,51-53] Although, in a discussion of the contracts set by 100 purchasing authorities for the year 1993/4, Redmayne et al showed that there was little indication of any fundamental shift from the historical pattern of resource distribution, they also found that some public health reports addressed the question of how to decide priorities. And although their report states that "the task of trying to re-shape the inherited pattern of priorities in the NHS. . . still appears to be tomorrow's agenda" (Redmayne et al,[46] p.7) there are also examples of health authorities who have chosen to set explicit criteria limiting or denying access to particular procedures. For example, eight authorities have limited cosmetic surgery, four have limited the treatment of asymptomatic wisdom teeth and eight have limited infertility treatment.[54]

There has been little direction provided by the UK Department of Health on this issue: indeed the Patient's Charter[48] is written in such a way that it denies limits on the finances available for health care [for example "Every citizen has the. . . rights: 1. to receive health care on the basis of clinical need. . .; 3. to receive emergency medical care at any time. . ." (Patient's Charter,[48] p.8)]. Instead, health authorities have been allowed to develop their own approaches to priority setting, with the inevitable result that some authorities have been innovative in their attempts to look at this issue explicitly, while others have not.[55] A recent report by the Health Select Committee of the House of Commons observed that "it is questionable whether the current national framework for priority setting provides adequate support to purchasers in taking decisions about the limits of local health services" (Health Committee,[55] p.lix). Although this statement implies an acceptance of explicit rationing for health care in the UK, the Government response is confusing.[19] In one paragraph there is the statement that ". . . budgets will always be finite while demand is potentially open-ended. There will always be a gap between all we wish to do and all that we can do. Setting priorities is a fact of life", (Government response to the first report from the Health Committee, Session 1994/5,[19] p.1) while in the next paragraph the response continues, "The Government's view is that the issue of rationing core services does not arise while there is scope for further improvements in effectiveness" (Government response to the first report from the Health Committee, Session 1994/5,[19] p.1). What this response fails to address is how a core service should be defined – and how priorities should be set between "non-core" services. The political and clinical reality is that implicit rationing is more comfortable. It is easier not to disrupt the status quo.

For politicians, explicit priority setting means that it is no longer possible to maintain the facade that there is no rationing of health care. For clinicians, whose ethical perspective has traditionally been individualistic, explicit priority setting means accepting the societal implications of choosing to treat particular individuals. Additionally, while clinicians might accept the idea of setting priorities in a general sense, they may be less willing to accept any of the services they themselves provide as anything less than a "priority".[56]

There will always be some individuals who lose as a result of changes in the allocation of resources, and this will undoubtedly be the result of priority setting in health care. Unless there is an acceptance of this fact, however, attempts to change the allocation of health care resources will forever run up against the problem of political backtracking. To maintain the deceit that there is no need to make choices, options for reducing services will be confined to those areas that are unable to command the attention of shroud-wavers. This is likely to be both inequitable and inefficient and will tend to maintain historical patterns of health care provision.

There is a question, however, as to whether implicit rationing, as well as being more acceptable politically and clinically, might also result in higher utility to society generally than explicit priority setting. The comment below was concerned with the Oregon plan, but it applies equally to all forms of explicit priority setting and emphasises the inherent difficulties in choosing explicitly to treat some individuals rather than others.

> The greatest source of anguish in the implementation of the plan will come in learning how to live with, and to rationalise, its failure to cover some people whose condition will pull at our sympathies. This anguish will be all the greater when the victims are visible and when

the accountability for their condition cannot be evaded. This is the greatest logical and emotional problem created by any set of priorities that set limits. We will, for one thing, always wonder if we are doing the right thing. We will always wonder, for another, if it might be possible to relieve the pain by some stratagem we have not yet devised. (Callahan,[57] p.85)

It may be that the utility that occurs to society is greater from implicit rationing than could be gained by having any of the following: an equitable system, a system that maximises the health improvement to society, or a democratic system in which lay preferences are considered alongside medical views. If the utility of pretending that there is no rationing in health care is greater than the potential utility that could be gained by setting priorities more explicitly, then perhaps implicit rationing should be maintained. It should not be maintained, however, if the main purpose it serves is to make the lives of politicians more comfortable. This is the feeling of many in the health service who "criticise the lack of courage in politicians who refuse to admit that rationing is a normal part of NHS life" (Hall,[58] p.3).

The remainder of this book is based on the assumption that implicit rationing is not likely to be more beneficial to society than setting priorities explicitly, and that some attempt should therefore be made to move towards explicit priority setting. A word should be said here, however, about the potential for implementing explicit priority setting in different cultural settings. It is likely that where incentives for change are stronger, explicit priority setting is more likely to succeed than in other settings. For example, the Oregon plan (discussed in detail in Chapter 2) has been implemented despite much opposition. In large part, this is a reflection of the extreme and apparent inequality in provision that existed before the plan was developed, combined with political leaders who were committed to change. Where there are not such obvious incentives, the implementation of explicit priority setting may be more difficult. The next section will continue with discussion of two opposing views about priority setting. The first concerns the overt technical rationing, which is, by many authors seen as "explicit" rationing. The second concerns a middle way: a form of explicit or rational rationing by the political process.

RELATED CHAPTERS

The discussion of implicit versus explicit rationing is related to the notion of individual versus societal ethics: if ethical considerations preclude clinicians from taking account of any but the individual currently receiving treatment, it is difficult to have anything but implicit rationing. Chapter 4 discusses in detail this question of individual versus societal ethics and its relationship to decisions about the allocation of scarce health care resources. The two case studies of rationing schemes presented in Chapters 2 and 3 provide an analysis of the progress from implicit to explicit rationing in Oregon and New Zealand.

EXPLICIT RATIONING BY POLITICAL PROCESSES OR METHODOLOGICAL TECHNIQUES?

There is a fundamental division between those advocating the more traditional view of explicit priority setting founded on specific principles and using particular methodologies to achieve these principles, and those advocating priority setting based on pluralistic bargaining, of whom the main proponent in the UK is Rudolf Klein. As with all the conflicts exposed in this chapter, and despite the rhetoric, in reality a combination of the two is most likely. The direction that each of the two schools of thought takes us in is, however, quite different, and two major sections of this book look at the different conflicts exposed by the two alternatives. For priority setting via bargaining processes, the tension between medical paternalism and lay participation becomes important, while the choice of a technical route lays bare the equity–efficiency conflict. In practice each conflict has relevance to both schools of thought, but is exposed with greater clarity in relation to one rather than the other. Before discussing these subsequent conflicts, however, the two alternatives will be described and compared.

A POLITICAL BASIS

A political basis for priority setting is founded on the idea that decisions about health care provision should be resolved through debate and bargaining.[46,59] Klein and colleagues feel that, because there is no obvious set of ethical principles or analytical tools that can be used by purchasing authorities (indeed they state that there are a "multiplicity of aims" which purchasers have to pursue[46]), the way in which priority setting can be made more rational is by concentrating on the processes and structures of decision-making.[59] Instead of searching for a specific principle upon which to base priorities, a system of bargaining should be used, whereby all bargainers bring their own objectives to the bargaining table. This does not mean implicit rationing, but instead a system whereby decisions are made explicitly and the reasoning behind, and justification for, specific judgements is clearly explained.[46,59] Klein believes that the objective of priority setting should be to build up the capacity to engage in such continuous and collective argument.[59] Such alternatives for health care rationing are variously referred to as "pluralistic bargaining", "incrementalism" and "muddling through elegantly".[9,59]

Who should be involved in this process of decision-making is left unclear by Klein, although he does state that "What is so often wrong about pluralistic bargaining is that it is not pluralistic enough: that discussion is dominated by some voices (notably those of the medical profession)" (Klein,[59] p.310). The question of lay participation in decision-making as opposed to the medical paternalism inevitably exhibited by implicit decision-making is of vital importance therefore in assessing whether pluralistic bargaining is an appropriate way forward in the rationing debate.

There are other aspects of pluralistic bargaining which are open to debate. There is an important distinction to be made between micro and macro level decision-making, and further questions about how broad allocations at the macro level are translated into clinical decisions at the micro level. Priority setting is not about making just one set of decisions, but is concerned with "the complex interaction of multiple decisions, taken at various levels in the organisation about allocating resources", (Klein,[59] p.309). This approach is quite different from the technical approach, which tends to assume that rules and methods are applicable across priority setting at different levels. For the purposes of pluralistic bargaining, therefore, there are also important questions about the level(s) of priority setting at which it is most important to have lay participation.[9]

A TECHNICAL BASIS

The development of technical frameworks for rationing has in large part been the preserve of health economics and public health medicine. Setting priorities on a technical basis assumes that a particular methodology will be chosen, based on a specific principle (or, less commonly, principles). Application of such a methodology will, then, assist in making decisions about which alternatives should be chosen. For example, some economists advocate the use of cost–utility analysis as a means of setting priorities. The costs of treatments for particular conditions are compared with the benefits in terms of quality-adjusted life-years (QALYs). The treatments which have the highest benefit per unit of cost are then the treatments which should be given priority. This is a technical solution in the sense that it involves a particular principle, maximising health gain, and a particular methodology, cost–utility analysis.

Such technical bases for priority setting do not tend to assume that there is a need to distinguish between different levels of priority setting. Instead it is assumed that by setting priorities across different conditions it is possible to aggregate backwards in order to set priorities, say, between specialties or between services.

Technical bases for priority setting are not only the preserve of economists, however. Other technical bases include the forms of priority setting based on equity – such as lotteries (not just a quirk as is often thought, but a policy with a substantial ethical basis), need-based rationing, and even age-based rationing. It is for this reason that, should a purchasing authority go down the technical route, the conflict between equity and efficiency is brought sharply into focus. These issues can, to some extent, be "fudged" by pluralistic bargaining, but they become very clear when alternative methodologies for priority setting are being chosen.

ADVANTAGES AND DISADVANTAGES OF THE TWO APPROACHES

The major advantage of a technical framework for priority setting, is that, not only are the decisions made explicit, but the objectives upon which these decisions are based are also made clear. If the objective of the purchasing authority is maximising "health gain" then plainly it can attempt to pursue this objective using, perhaps, the technique of cost–utility analysis (see Chapter 5). Use of such technical frameworks may move the health service closer to specified objectives such as efficiency or equity than a system of pluralistic bargaining may be able to do. A kind of neutrality, in which priorities are set free of political interference or clinical dominance, is also implied, and for many the use of such technical methodologies is an "easy option" in that the methodology is readily available and has been previously used.

These potential advantages over pluralistic bargaining may, however, be unrealised. The search for elegance in priority setting may prove elusive: what looks like a sound methodology may be completely impractical. A huge quantity of data is often required for technical methods of priority setting. These data may include the costs of interventions, the effectiveness of interventions, the extent of illness in a population, and, possibly, information about public preferences. A common problem is that these extensive quantities of data are often simply not available, particularly given the heterogeneity of patients. There may also be methodological weaknesses and inherent value judgements in the techniques, of which non-experts may be unaware. It is claimed that rationing by the political process, on the other hand, is "ideally suited to situations of extreme uncertainty and complexity where information is poor and incomplete" (Hunter,[9] p.28).

Added to the data problems for technical rationing may be greater difficulties in implementing the results of technical priority setting. Pluralistic bargaining, on the other hand, implies that at the end of the bargaining process a decision will have been reached. This decision will usually be based on compromise and, because it has been reached by the bargaining parties, it may have a greater chance of implementation than a decision which has been taken primarily on the basis of a particular principle. This is particularly the case given that the policy and funding structures of health care may not relate closely to any of the "techniques" for priority setting on the basis of equity or efficiency. With both forms of priority setting, however, there are issues about how to get right the incentives for implementing priorities once they have been defined.

With pluralistic bargaining there are fundamental questions concerning *who* should be involved in the bargaining process and indeed how this decision should be made. Who is included in the bargaining process may have huge implications for the subsequent priorities. Where the groups included are limited, there is a danger that such bargaining might slip back into implicit priority setting without anyone really noticing.

The reality is that neither option alone will fulfil the requirements of explicit priority setting. Technical methods will never be able to deal with the entire health service budget, but priority setting via political processes should ideally utilise the sort of information on effectiveness, efficiency, need and equity provided by technical methods as a basis for bargaining. Inevitably both elements will be involved in priority setting. It is a question of the extent to which each is used and the respective emphasis on these different alternatives.

Each of the conflicts exposed by these two traditions will now be considered, beginning with the equity–efficiency conflict and its relationship to technical rationing.

RELATED CHAPTERS

The two case studies of rationing schemes presented in Chapters 2 and 3 were chosen for their different bases in technical priority setting and priority setting by bargaining methods. The two case studies thus provide a contrast between these two forms of rationing. Chapter 4, which looks at the ethical basis for priority setting, also relates to the choice between approaches in its discussion of the differences between health economists, who tend to prefer technical approaches, and health workers, who tend to be very suspicious of the technical alternatives. In the final chapter of the book a way forward for priority setting is proposed. The framework for priority setting discussed in this chapter explicitly aims to combine the two approaches of technical priority setting and pluralistic bargaining.

TECHNICAL PRIORITY SETTING: THE EQUITY–EFFICIENCY CONFLICT

There are many different precise principles which could be used as the basis for technical models of priority setting: for example, maximising health gain, equalising access to treatment for those of equal need, or equalising treatment by age. The majority, however, fit into the two broad areas of equity and efficiency.

The notion of efficiency is based on a maximising concept: the idea that it is possible to maximise the total amount of "benefit" available in the community if both the costs and benefits of an intervention are considered. It thus pursues a utilitarian ethic of the greatest good for the greatest number, and generally assumes that the distribution of this good is not an important issue. The principle of efficiency is generally to be found in the models advocated by health economists, but in very few others. Models based on the principle of efficiency are discussed in Chapter 5.

Equity principles are concerned with just distribution. Equity as a concept is less precise than efficiency and has more variants. For example, all models that are ostensibly based on "need", however this is defined, are essentially concerned with equity (e.g. equal health care for equal need, equal access for equal need, etc.), as are many other models which have been put forward, such as equal treatment for those of equal age,[60,61] and equal treatment for all based on a lottery.[62–64] Priority setting techniques based on equity principles are discussed in Chapter 6.

Priorities based on equity, however defined, will almost certainly conflict with those based on efficiency. A stark illustration of this conflict appears in a paper by Gaston et al.[65] This paper was concerned with access to cadaveric kidneys for renal transplant candidates. HLA matching improves the rate of graft survival and

10
20

thus improves the efficiency of renal transplant. Matching by HLA was the prevailing policy for deciding who should receive a graft. This policy was found to have had a negative impact on black patients for whom there is less likely to be a match. Pursuing the most efficient policy in terms of health gain therefore has costs in equity, which the authors of this paper believed to be unjustified. This paper illustrates a tension between racial equity and efficiency: to increase equity in provision, diminished efficiency must be accepted. Such tensions will almost certainly occur between any equity basis for priority setting and efficiency (and indeed between different equity bases and between different efficiency bases). [The paper by Gaston et al, however, does not illustrate a conflict between efficiency and equal treatment for those with equal ability to benefit. This is because the only "cost" discussed here is the cost of a kidney. If other costs were included, however, there would almost certainly have been conflict noted between these two principles.] Much of the discussion of particular techniques for priority setting is focused on this conflict rather than problems or difficulties with the particular techniques. For example, the development of the QALY methodology and its use in cost–utility analysis, based on efficiency, has resulted in criticism on the basis of the resulting inequality in treatment for people of different ages.[66–68]

For purchasing authorities anticipating the use of a technical framework for priority setting, clarity of understanding regarding the ethical bases of particular methodologies is essential (see Chapter 4). The use of a particular methodology is only justified if it will result in priorities based on the desired objective. Although Chapters 5 and 6 describe in detail a number of methodologies based on either efficiency or equity, there are few, if any, adequate methods for making trade-offs between one principle and another. Just as basing priorities on single different principles will result in different sets of priorities, basing priorities on multiple principles will result in different priorities depending on whether each principle is given an equal role (however defined!) or some principles are allowed to take a more dominant role.

The likely reality of the efficiency–equity conflict is that priorities will encompass both principles. If efficiency is pursued to the exclusion of equity there may well be substantial sectors of society who do not receive treatment. This is likely to be considered to be unfair, and thus unacceptable both politically and publicly. However, if equity is pursued without regard to efficiency some people may receive highly resource-intensive treatments at the expense of others who could be treated at a fraction of the cost. Again this is unlikely to be acceptable.

RELATED CHAPTERS

The main related chapters are those examining in detail the methods proposed for priority setting which have their basis in equity principles (Chapter 6) and efficiency principles (Chapter 5). However, further discussion of this conflict also appears in Chapters 2 and 3 (looking at the use of these principles made in Oregon and New Zealand) and Chapter 4 (the ethical basis for the equity–efficiency conflict). In Chapter 9 the problem of trading off one principle against another is discussed in more detail. This chapter also proposes a way forward for priority setting which incorporates both principles.

POLITICAL BARGAINING: MEDICAL PATERNALISM AND LAY PARTICIPATION

The involvement, or not, of different groups of individuals in the pluralistic bargaining process is likely to have huge implications for the chosen priorities. The conflict arises in its broadest sense over the question of whether or not the "public" should be involved. Beyond that issue are many other conflicts: what is meant by lay participation? who should be asked to participate – who are the "public"? who should decide who participates? how should lay views be incorporated into the bargaining process? what weight should different views be accorded? These are the sorts of difficult and fundamental questions that lie behind easy assertions that the public should be consulted. On the other hand, pluralistic bargaining is pluralistic no longer if the only involvement comes from the medical and associated professions.

There is no real history of lay participation in the NHS. In fact there has been a steady erosion of lay control of the provision of health care since the nineteenth century and the creation, via the welfare state, of a laity whose defining characteristic is that it stands *outside* authority over health care provision (see Chapter 7). Neither are there academic theories that support the acquisition of public preferences. Until the 1980s (with the exception of the appointed Community Health Councils) the public was largely excluded from NHS policy making. It is quite clear, however, that allowing the public a say in the sorts of health services that they receive is becoming *de rigueur*. Although a number of government publications have stressed individuals' rights as consumers (e.g. the government white paper, *Working for patients*, 1989,[47] aimed to put "the needs of patients first" whilst *The Patients' Charter*,[69] published by the Department of Health in 1992, set out a number of rights for patients being treated under the NHS), others have stressed the desire for acquiring a lay view about priorities.[19,70] Even the Patients' Charter re-enforced the need for health authorities to seek people's views and to provide better information about health and health services.[69] *Local Voices*,[70] the NHS Management Executive paper published in 1992, has provided the fullest explanation of the intention to incorporate people's views into the NHS, but the general desire to involve the public had not diminished in 1995 when the Health Committee report *Priority Setting in the NHS: Purchasing* recommended that "Health authorities must be able to demonstrate, for example. . . that input from local people has influenced change to the purchasing agenda and the planning of services" (Health Committee,[55] p.lv).

The conflict between medical paternalism and lay participation is not as simple to resolve as one might think. After all, who wants paternalism? But do lay people want to have a say in the priorities attached to different forms of health care that are provided for them? The answers to these questions are not self-evident. There are arguments both for including and excluding the public.

Let us first consider the advantages of incorporating a lay viewpoint. To a large extent these advantages are concerned with the changes in service provision that might result. Priorities set in this way will reflect what people want, including their preferences, concerns and values. By incorporating public preferences into pluralistic bargaining the resulting services may be better suited to local needs. Not only will there be such practical benefits from public participation, however, there will also be the advantage that the whole bargaining process will become more explicit. The public will be able to influence the choices that are made and change decisions that they do not agree with. There is a question, however, concerning what the lay viewpoint actually consists of. Lay views may most properly come from random samples of individuals, but they may also be provided by interested individuals or community representatives.

There is support for incorporating public views from a number of public bodies who traditionally favour the consumer. The Association of Community Health Councils of England and Wales states that

> It is not acceptable for these decisions to be taken secretly without the opportunity for public debate. (Memorandum submitted by the Association of Community Health Councils of England and Wales (PS74), Health Committee,[71] p.171)

whilst the National Consumer Council makes clear its opinion that the public should not bear the responsibility for setting priorities:

> consumers have a vital role to play in informing all aspects of policy-making in the NHS. However, we do not believe that consumers should be responsible for priority setting itself. (Memorandum submitted by the National Consumer Council (PS124), Health Committee,[54] p.210).

Let us now consider the alternative viewpoint. It is hard to argue against the platitude that "the public" should be included in planning health services. In many cases, however, decisions are controversial, even unpalatable. In fact, considering the history of lay participation in the NHS, (see Chapter 7) it would be fair to say that it seems unlikely that the public would have been invited to contribute if the issues facing the NHS had not been difficult and unpleasant! There is a serious question as to whether the public could, or should, be forced to make unpalatable judgements, such as between the old and young, deserving and not. Inevitably, such decisions tap prejudices and preconceptions, and people's views are shaped by the media and by the mode of presentation. Opening up the can of issues surrounding priorities may release a number of unpleasant worms. There may be talk of the deserving and the undeserving. Groups may become singled out for having treatment withheld: those deemed incapable of benefit, such as the infirm, elderly or disabled. It would not then be an enormous step to single out other disadvantaged groups, such as the unemployed, or the "intentionally" sick (alcoholics, the obese). Asked to choose between cases or categories of patients, the public will inevitably be swayed by emotional consideration. Shroud wavers may triumph over those seeking dull but incrementally effective treatments.

These issues are emotive and easily overdrawn, but involving public preferences may not result in a more effective and efficient health service. It is unclear whether services chosen by the local public will necessarily be "appropriate" on the basis of, for example, epidemiological evidence. There is at least a possibility that the public will wish to emphasise high-technology medicine at the expense of less "glamorous" forms of care, and there is the problem that "hot topics" in the media may acquire greater priority purely because of greater interest in, and knowledge about, these issues.

This leads on to a further important question concerning the seriousness with which health authorities are willing to incorporate preferences which might be different from their own. Is there genuine support for incorporating the lay view in health care decision-making, or is this expressed support merely an attempt to support medical paternalism, albeit paternalism from a different group of medics? *Local Voices* states that one of the reasons for purchasers to obtain public views is to enhance their credibility in negotiations with providers.[70] It is suggested that purchasers are likely to be more persuasive and successful in their negotiations if they secure public support. This could mean that purchasing authorities merely co-opt public views to support their own policies, or it may indicate a deeper willingness to include the public. Are public views being sought in order to bring their views to the bargaining table, or is the aim to bolster the public health viewpoint? The answer to this question is not clear. There is a particular conflict where, at a local scale, public preferences directly contradict national policy. It is not clear what health authorities should, or would, do then – argue for national policies, or implement local preferences?

The question of whether there should be lay participation in health care decision-making is a thorny one. It is also a question to which little attention has been paid. It is much easier to debate the minutiae of how participation should be achieved than to discuss the conflict that arises between paternalism and participation. To say that the public should be excluded from the decision-making process implies that those with medical training or administrative experience should continue as they have since the NHS began, with implicit and unspoken priorities. To include the public may not only distress them, but may also result in a greater degree of intolerance. David Hunter states that "effective public involvement in rationing decisions ought to be encouraged where, and in ways that are, appropriate but it needs to be buttressed and supported. . ." (Hunter,[9] 1993, p.28). Major questions remain, however. There is a question over the real willingness of purchasers to incorporate the views and opinions of the public, and, if this is achieved, how far they will go in changing existing services to meet the priorities expressed by "the public". There is also a question over the willingness of members of the public to participate in difficult decisions about priority setting in health care.

RELATED CHAPTERS

Extensive discussion of the history of lay participation in the NHS is to be found in Chapter 7. The controversies over how best to incorporate information about a lay viewpoint are discussed in Chapter 8, as are practical methods of acquiring information about public preferences. Additionally, Chapters 2 and 3 look at the ways in which information about public preferences has been incorporated into the priority setting exercises in New Zealand and Oregon.

CONCLUSION

There are many available paths through the rationing maze – all of which are imperfect. This chapter has provided a structure for viewing the different positions and analysing the tensions between them. In this chapter, as in the rest of the book, the aim has not been to advocate one approach at the expense of all others: each view offers insights into this complex area and the debate is not yet so far advanced that it can afford to ignore any of the contributions offered.

Indeed, as yet, there has been little public debate about the rationing of health care. What debate exists is not aided by the sensationalist approach to limitations in the funding for health care taken by the media.[9] Unless, however, like ostriches, we prefer to hide our collective heads in the sand by pretending that these limits do not exist, sustained public debate is required.

Health care priority setting is an elaborate and intricate issue, and it is clear that the many issues it inspires cannot be solved by the production of a single document such as this – even were such a "solution" possible. Be reassured, however, that the book does not comprise a pessimistic or despairing view of the potential for priority setting in health care. Rather, it supports a more positive view. While acknowledging the conflicts, the complexity and the confusion, there is also the recognition that choices can be made about how we proceed. There can undoubtedly be debate about how resources should be allocated; there can almost certainly be improvements in the allocation of resources. Priority setting does not require perfection, but merely improvement. The final chapter of the book offers a compromise – one way forward (but certainly not the only way) – which attempts to combine the disciplinary approaches offered by those practising in the area of social medicine: epidemiologists, health economists, medical sociologists and political scientists.

REFERENCES

1. Anon. Who should live, who should die? *Which* 1994; **July**: 50–3.
2. Hall C, Mackinnon I. Cancer girl loses fight for treatment. *The Independent* 1995; **11 March**: 1.
3. Khalid MI. Access to heart surgery for smokers: denying treatment is indefensible. *BMJ* 1993; **306**: 1408.
4. Mamode N. Access to heart surgery for smokers: denying access more

costly. *BMJ* 1993; **306**: 1408.
5. Vithayathil E, Michael A. Access to heart surgery for smokers: the NHS can't treat only saints. *BMJ* 1993; **306**: 1408–9.
6. Grant SCD, Bennett DH, Bray CL, Brooks NH, Levy RD, Ward C. Access to heart surgery for smokers: each patient a special case. *BMJ* 1993; **306**: 1408.
7. Odom NJ, Ashraf SS, Sharif MH, Akhtar K. Access to heart surgery for smokers: persuade smokers to give up before surgery. *BMJ* 1993; **307**: 128.
8. Mooney G, Gerard K, Donaldson C, Farrar S. *Priority setting in purchasing. Some practical guidelines.* NAHAT, Birmingham, 1992.
9. Hunter D. *Rationing dilemmas in healthcare.* NAHAT, Birmingham, 1993.
10. Alberti G, Tudor Hart J. Rational care needed, not rationing. *BMJ* 1993; **306**: 1072.
11. Hershfield NB. Rationing health care services. *Can Med Assoc J* 1988; **139**: 9.
12. Relman AS. The trouble with rationing. *N Engl J Med* 1990; **323**(13): 911–13.
13. Wolfe PR. Health care rationing. *Science* 1990; **247**: 661.
14. Relman AS. Is rationing inevitable? *N Engl J Med* 1990; **322**(25): 1809–10.
15. Honigsbaum F. Rationing health care. *BMJ* 1991; **302**: 288–9.
16. Robinson EL. The Oregon Basic Health Services Act – a model for state reform. *Vanderbilt Law Review* 1992; **45**(4): 977–1014.
17. Reagan MD. Health care rationing. What does it mean? *N Engl J Med* 1988; **319**(17): 1149–51.
18. Aaron HJ, Schwarz WB. *The painful prescription. Rationing hospital care.* The Brookings Institution, Washington, 1984.
19. Department of Health. *Government response to the first report from the Health Committee session 1994–95.* HMSO, London, 1995.
20. Government Committee on Choices in Health Care. *Choices in health care.* Ministry of Welfare, Health and Cultural Affairs, Rijswijk, 1992.
21. National Advisory Committee on Core Health and Disability Support Services. *The best of health. Deciding on the health services we value most.* Department of Health, Wellington, New Zealand, 1992.
22. Groves T. Public disagrees with professionals over NHS rationing. *BMJ* 1993; **306**: 673.
23. Secretary of State for Health. *Priority setting in the Health Service.* Speech to BMA/King's Fund/Patients Association, 11 March 1993. Also: Brindle D. Some NHS treatment 'must go'. *The Guardian* 1995; **29 March**: 10.
24. US Department of Health and Human Services. Personal Health Care Expenditures: 1992 Highlights. *Health Care Financing Review 1995; Medicare and Medicaid Statistical Supplement*: 1.

25. Callahan D. *What kind of life. The limits of medical progress.* Simon and Schuster, New York, 1990.
26. Callahan D. Rationing medical progress. The way to affordable health care. *N Engl J Med* 1990; **322**(25): 1810–13.
27. Frankel SJ. Health needs, health-care requirements, and the myth of infinite demand. *Lancet* 1991; **337**: 1588–90.
28. *The concise Oxford dictionary of current English.* Oxford University Press, Oxford, 1982.
29. *New Collins concise English dictionary.* William Collins, Glasgow, 1982.
30. Klein R. Rationing health care. *BMJ* 1984; **289**: 143–4.
31. Rooks JP. Let's admit we ration health care – then set priorities. *Am J Nurs* 1990; **90**(6): 39–43.
32. Fox DM, Leichter HM. Rationing care in Oregon: the new accountability. *Health Affairs* 1991; **Summer**: 7–27.
33. Eddy DM. What's going on in Oregon? *J Am Med Assoc* 1991; **266**(3): 417–20.
34. Smith R. Crisis in American health care. *BMJ* 1990; **300**: 765–6.
35. Aaron H, Schwarz WB. Rationing health care: the choice before us. *Science* 1990; **247**: 418–22.
36. McGuire A, Henderson J, Mooney G. *The economics of health care. An introductory text.* Routledge & Kegan Paul, London, 1988.
37. Crawshaw R. Health care rationing. *Science* 1990; **247**: 662–3.
38. Grimes DS. Rationing health care. *Lancet* 1987; **i**: 615–16.
39. Wiener JM. Rationing in America: overt and covert. In: Strosberg MA, Weiner JM, Baker R, Fein IA, eds. *Rationing America's medical care: the Oregon plan and beyond.* The Brookings Institution, Washington, DC, 1992: 12–23.
40. Dean M. Is your treatment economic, effective, efficient? *Lancet* 1991; **337**: 480–1.
41. Parsons V. Rationing: at the cutting edge. *BMJ* 1991; **303**: 1553.
42. Smith R. Rationing: the search for sunlight. *BMJ* 1991; **303**: 1561–2.
43. Baker R. The inevitability of health care rationing: a case study of rationing in the British National Health Service. In: Strosberg MA, Weiner JM, Baker R, Fein IA, eds. *Rationing America's medical care: the Oregon plan and beyond.* The Brookings Institution, Washington, DC, 1992: 208–29.
44. Roland M. General Practitioners' referral rates. *BMJ* 1988; **297**: 437–8.
45. Wilkin D. Patterns of referral: explaining variation. In: Roland M, Coulter A, eds. *Hospital referrals.* Oxford University Press, Oxford, 1992: 76–91.
46. Redmayne S, Klein R, Day P. *Sharing out resources. Purchasing and priority setting in the NHS.* NAHAT, Birmingham, 1993.

47. Department of Health. *Working for patients*. HMSO, London, 1989.
48. Department of Health. *The patient's charter*. HMSO, London, 1992.
49. Maynard A. Priorities in nether Netherland. *Health Service J* 1992; **27 Aug**: 19.
50. Meek C. Pie in the sky. Can healthcare rationing ever be objective? *BMA News Rev* 1992; **September**: 15–17.
51. Klein R, Redmayne S. *Patterns of priorities. A study of the purchasing and rationing policies of health authorities*. NAHAT, Birmingham, 1992.
52. Ham C. Health care rationing. *BMJ* 1995; **310**: 1483–4.
53. Mechanic D. Dilemmas in rationing health care services: the case for implicit rationing. *BMJ* 1995; **310**: 1655–9.
54. National Consumer Council. Memorandum submitted by the National Consumer Council (PS124). In: Health Committee, ed. *Priority setting in the NHS: purchasing. Volume II. Minutes of evidence and appendices*. HMSO, London, 1995: 210–16.
55. Health Committee. *Priority setting in the NHS: purchasing. Volume I*. HMSO, London, 1995.
56. Wight J. Rationing of health care in medicine. *J R Coll Phys London* 1993; **27**(2): 175–6.
57. Callahan D. Ethics and priority setting in Oregon. *Health Affairs* 1991; **Summer**: 78–87.
58. Hall C. Policy issues cloud decisions over treatment. *The Independent* 1995; **11 March**: 3.
59. Klein R. Dimensions of rationing: who should do what? *BMJ* 1993; **307**: 309–11.
60. Callahan D. *Setting limits. Medical goals in an aging society*. Simon and Schuster, New York, 1987.
61. Jecker NS. Age-based rationing and women. *J Am Med Assoc* 1991; **266**(21): 3012–15.
62. Kilner JF. *Who lives? Who dies? Ethical criteria in patient selection*. Yale University Press, New Haven, 1990.
63. Hope T, Sprigings D, Crisp R. "Not clinically indicated": patients' interests or resource allocation? *BMJ* 1993; **306**: 379–81.
64. Broome J. Fairness versus doing the most good. *Hastings Center Report* 1994; **July–August**: 36–9.
65. Gaston RS, Ayres I, Dooley LG, Diethelm AG. Racial equity in renal transplantation. The disparate impact of HLA-based allocation. *J Am Med Assoc* 1993; **270**(11): 1352–6.
66. Grimley Evans J. Quality of life assessments and elderly people. In: Hopkins A, ed. *Measures of the quality of life*. Royal College of Physicians, London, 1992: 107–16.
67. Smith A, Maynard A, Grimley Evans J, Harris J. The ethics of resource

allocation. Proceedings of a symposium held at the University of Manchester during the 33rd Annual Scientific Meeting of the Society for Social Medicine, September 1989. *J Epidemiol Commun Health* 1990; **44**: 187–90.

68. Grimley Evans J. Age and equality. *Ann NY Acad Sci* 1988; **530**: 118–24.

69. Anon. The Patient's Charter. *NHSME News* 1991; **50**: 1–2.

70. NHS Management Executive. *Local voices. The views of local people in purchasing for health*. Department of Health, London, 1992.

71. Association of Community Health Councils of England and Wales. Memorandum submitted by the Association of Community Health Councils of England and Wales (PS74). In: Health Committee, ed. *Priority setting in the NHS: purchasing. Volume II. Minutes of evidence and appendices*. HMSO, London, 1995: 171–7.

PART TWO

From Implicit to Explicit Rationing: Two Steps Forward and One Step Back

CHAPTER TWO

JOANNA COAST

The Oregon Plan: Technical Priority Setting in the USA

One particular attempt to allocate priorities to the whole spectrum of health care has generated a huge amount of interest in the arena of priority setting: the Oregon plan. In 1989 the state of Oregon began work on devising a list of conditions and treatments, with those conditions and treatments with the highest priority at the top of the list, and those conditions with the lowest priority at the bottom of the list. Those proposing the scheme wished to offer a basic health service package which covers services with the highest priority, by drawing a cut-off at a particular point on the list and funding all services which lie above this line and refusing funding for all services below the line.

The Oregon plan was the first large-scale attempt to derive a set of priorities to cover all possible health interventions, and has affected the level of ambition with which those responsible for making decisions about health care are attempting to set priorities. It has also challenged the belief that health care can, and should, be an unlimited benefit.[1]

The chapter begins by discussing a forerunner to the Oregon plan, Oregon Health Decisions. The details and history of the Oregon plan are described in the second section of the chapter, and the final part of the chapter is a discussion of the success of the plan. This discussion relates in large part to the conflicts identified in Chapter 1.

Priority Setting: The Health Care Debate.
Edited by J. Coast, J. Donovan and S. Frankel. © 1996 John Wiley & Sons Ltd.

OREGON HEALTH DECISIONS, 1987–1989

Oregon Health Decisions, a network of citizens aiming to raise awareness of bioethical problems among the public, began a project called "Oregon health priorities for the 1990s" in 1987.[2] During the project 19 community meetings were held across the state of Oregon. The community meetings attempted to attract the general public to attend, and direct mailings, newspaper articles, radio advertising and civic organisations were used to attract people to the meetings.[2]

In these meetings individuals were asked to discuss priority setting at different levels of health care. Initially individuals were asked to consider the priority that health care should receive in comparison to other social needs (69% favoured higher expenditure on health services).[2] Secondly, individuals were asked to consider what general priorities should be assigned within the health care sector: given a matrix of 16 "health care building blocks" individuals were asked to assign high priority to five, medium priority to six and low priority to five. The matrix contained four categories on each axis: one axis was for point in the life-cycle (infants, children, adults and elderly); the other axis was for different types of health care (critical, long-term, short-term and preventive). No information is provided regarding the reasons for these particular choices. The five categories given high priority were Critical–Children, Long-term–Elderly, Preventive–Infants, Preventive–Children and Preventive–Adults. The five categories for which priority was considered low were Critical–Elderly, Long-term–Infants, Long-term–Children, Short-term–Elderly, Preventive–Elderly.[2]

Following these community meetings, in September 1988, 50 delegates (including 24 participants from the community meetings) met as a "Citizen's Health Care Parliament". At this parliament, 15 principles were passed as resolutions, including one resolution, number 11, which states that "Allocation of health resources should be based, in part, on a scale of public attitudes that quantifies the trade-off between length of life and quality of life" (Crawshaw et al,[2] p.445). The full set of principles was then published and sent to all state legislators. Many of the principles established by the Health Care Parliament are now reflected in Oregon's Senate Bills 27 and 935 (see below).[2]

THE OREGON PLAN

The most ambitious attempt yet at setting priorities for health care has been undertaken in Oregon in the USA. In the USA there is a conflict between providing largely unlimited care for a proportion of those patients unable to purchase health care insurance, i.e. those eligible for Medicaid, and providing a lesser degree of cover for a broader base of patients. The Oregon plan is an attempt to resolve this conflict using an essentially technical basis for explicit rationing.

Oregon's priority-setting exercise was a direct response to a previous, more painful attempt at altering the accepted priorities of the Medicaid system in Oregon. In 1987, the Joint Ways and Means Committee of the Oregon legislature voted to discontinue funding for organ transplantation (liver, bone marrow, pancreas and heart) and instead to include a further 1500 individuals in Medicaid coverage for basic health care, including antenatal care.[3] (The decision to discontinue funding for organ transplants has, however, been stated to have been unrelated at the time to decisions to increase antenatal funding.[4]) The discontinued organ transplantation programme was projected to affect 34 patients over the following two years. Previous experience in Oregon had suggested that transplantations were marked by limited success among relatively few recipients, and by great expense.[3] No public debate was involved in the decision and little immediate reaction followed.[3]

As a result of the decision, a seven-year-old boy, Coby Howard, was denied funding for a bone marrow transplant for leukaemia. He died when his private fund was US$30 000 short of the US$100 000 total needed for transplantation.[5] Although two adults had previously also been refused transplants under the same policy, they had attracted little media attention in comparison.[3] The reaction which followed the death of Coby Howard and the resulting media coverage forced the federal government to order, from 1 April 1990, the restoration of transplants across the nation for those under 21 years of age.[6] It was this first, perhaps naïve, attempt to set priorities in health care that led Oregon, already toying with the idea of priority setting through its Oregon Health Decisions programme, towards a full priority-setting exercise across all conditions and treatments.

The Oregon plan was, therefore, conceived as a solution to a particular problem facing the state regarding the widening of health care insurance to individuals presently uninsured either privately or through the federal Medicaid system, whilst remaining within a fixed budget. In the words of two commentators, the state of Oregon was faced with the dilemma of "all for some or some for all" (Street and Richardson,[7] p.127). At the time the Oregon experiment began the state's Medicaid eligibility level was 58% of the federal poverty level,[8] and approximately 450 000 Oregonians were estimated to have no health coverage.[9] It was estimated early in 1990 that approximately 120 000 new Medicaid recipients would be admitted to the Medicaid scheme by 1995 as a direct result of expanding eligibility to all those with family incomes below the federal poverty line.[10] It was also estimated that 97% of Oregon's population would have insurance coverage as a result of the new Oregon plan.[11]

In 1989 the Oregon senate passed three pieces of legislation known as the Oregon Basic Health Services Act. Senate Bill 27 directed the Oregon Health Services Commission to form a prioritised health service list to determine the treatments which would be funded for a particular group of those receiving Medicaid. Senate Bill 27 also mandated an increase in the coverage of Medicaid from 51% (depending on category of aid) to 100% of the federal poverty level.[12] The bill was passed in conjunction with two others which aimed to widen further the coverage of those presently uninsured. Senate Bill 935 required all employers to offer health insurance to their workers by 1994, and Senate Bill 534 established a risk pool for the coverage of persons who were uninsurable because of pre-existing conditions.[12]

The Oregon Health Services Commission began the task of forming a priority list in the autumn of 1989. It began the priority-setting process by reviewing a number of methods for, and approaches to, priority setting. Three subcommittees were initially formed: the Social Values Subcommittee with the aim of obtaining information about public preferences; the Health Outcomes Subcommittee to seek an objective system to measure the effectiveness of treatment and to develop a benefit analysis and cost–utility analysis; and the Mental Health Care and Chemical Dependency Subcommittee to assist the Commission with prioritisation of mental health care and chemical dependency services (MHCD).[12]

The Commission initially concluded that the best available method for prioritisation was the use of "cost–benefit with a quality of life component" (Oregon Health Services Commission,[12] p.15). This method was also to involve the use of social valuations. The method will be referred to as cost–utility analysis from this point as this coincides more closely with the usual economic terminology.[13] [In cost–utility analysis QALYs are usually used (as a measure of health-related utility) as a measure of outcome. In cost–benefit analysis the measure of outcome is valued in monetary terms.]

The work began with the formation of condition/treatment pairs in which the diagnosis and appropriate treatment were noted. Conditions were segregated using the diagnostic ICD-9 and DSM-III-R codes, and treatments were segregated using CPT-4 treatment codes. Examples of condition/treatment pairs include "Acute Myocardial Infarction/Medical Treatment" and "Hernia without Obstruction or Gangrene/Repair".[12] All condition/treatment pairs were then ranked according to the public valuation of the improvement in health gain per unit of cost, with those conditions with the greatest benefit per unit of cost at the top of the list.

Public preferences (social values) were obtained through public hearings, community meetings and a telephone survey, although no attempt was made to rate specific conditions because it was felt that the public did not have the competence to make such judgements.[6] The telephone survey was developed to collect public values for particular symptoms and levels of functional impairment associated with illness. These values were then fed into the Quality of Well-Being Scale[14,15] and linked with information about the outcomes of particular treatments for particular conditions to derive utilities.

Information about health outcomes was based on an age-cohort approach to measuring treatment effectiveness for given diagnoses.[12] Collection of outcomes data began with an attempt to review medical research literature, but "It became apparent this approach was unwieldy and counterproductive because of the 'shelf-life' of the data and a lack of conclusive studies of effectiveness" (Oregon Health Services Commission,[12] p.10). Judgements by providers of health care were therefore used to obtain information about treatment effectiveness and health outcomes. This information was then combined with information about costs to develop a prioritised list of health services ranked according to the relevant utility per unit of cost. Costs were assessed using charge categories, rather than specific dollar costs for treatment of each condition. No attempt was made to assess the costs associated with non-treatment.[12]

The first version of the Oregon priority list, ranking approximately 1600 medical procedures, was produced on 2 May 1990.[5] Harvey Klevit, a member of the Oregon Health Services Commission, has been quoted as saying that he "looked at the first two pages of that list and threw it in the trash can" (Morell,[16] p.468). The first list was immediately abandoned because of its counterintuitive ordering of condition/treatment pairs, and "the presence of numerous flaws, aberrations and errors" (Klevit et al,[5] p.915). The reasons for the failure of this first list were judged to be the failure of cost–utility analysis to provide an acceptable ordering[17] and the poor quality of data incorporated into the model[5,9] (see below, however).

For the second list the reliance on cost–utility analysis was abandoned, and instead the list was formed using a three-step methodology.[12] In the first instance, health service categories were created and ranked (using a ranked categorisation method recommended by Hadorn[17]). The second step of the process involved ranking condition/treatment pairs, within categories, according to the net benefit produced by treatment. Finally, Commission judgement was used to make adjustments to the prioritised list of health services.[12] Each of these steps is described below.

The first step of the methodology involved forming health service categories and ranking these. Seventeen categories were formed and were ranked from most to least important.[12] Table 2.1 shows the seventeen categories in the order in which they were ranked. The categories were ranked by the Commissioners. Each Commissioner gave a relative weight to each category from 0 to 100 for each of three attributes: "value to society", "value to an individual at risk of needing the service" and "essential to a basic health care package". These attributes are reflections of the values expressed in the 47 community meetings. A modified Delphi technique was used to assist the commission in arriving at a consensus.[12] Particular condition/treatment pairs were then assigned to specific categories according to (a) whether the condition was acute or chronic, (b) the

Table 2.1   Ranked categorisation of health services (ranked from most to least important)[12]

1 Acute Fatal	Treatment prevents death with full recovery
2 Maternity Care	Including disorders of the newborn
3 Acute Fatal	Treatment prevents death without full recovery
4 Preventive Care for Children	
5 Chronic Fatal	Treatment improves life-span and quality of life
6 Reproductive Services	Excludes maternity and fertility services
7 Comfort Care	Palliative therapy for conditions in which death is imminent
8 Preventive Dental Care	Adults and children
9 Proven Effective Preventive Care for Adults	
10 Acute Non-fatal	Treatment causes return to health status
11 Chronic Non-fatal	One-time treatment improves quality of life
12 Acute Non-fatal	Treatment without return to previous health state
13 Chronic Non-fatal	Repetitive treatment improves quality of life
14 Acute Non-fatal	Treatment expediates recovery of self-limiting condition
15 Infertility Services	
16 Less Effective Preventive Care for Adults	
17 Fatal or Non-fatal	Treatment causes minimal or no improvement in quality of life

degree of fatality (where fatality was defined as a chance of death without treatment of 1% or more), and (c) the improvement in quality of life.[12]

The net benefit assigned to each condition/treatment pair was calculated using both public preferences (as obtained during the telephone survey) and information about the outcomes likely to result from treatment as specified by health care providers. Net benefit was based on the average patient with median age at onset and a blend of outcome probabilities, with a frame for assessment of five years subsequent to treatment.[12] Buist refers to the subsequent measure as the "net quality adjusted survival rate after 5 years" (Buist,[18] p.21).

For the telephone survey, random telephone calls were made throughout Oregon. In all 1001 telephone surveys were completed, with a completion rate of 23.3%.[12] The refusal rate for completion was also 23.3%, with the remaining 53.4% of calls not being completed for reasons of disconnection, no answer, business or government telephone number, midway termination of the survey, language barrier, answering machines and numbers not tried.[12] Households below the poverty line were undersampled, and the white population was oversampled.[12] Respondents were asked to rate 31 health states with values from 0 ("as bad as death") to 100 ("good health"). These then provided values for the public of Oregon to be used with a modified Quality of Well-Being Scale developed by Robert Kaplan.[19] The Quality of Well-Being Scale had not previously been used on such a large scale, but had been used in small clinical trials.[20]

The information about public preferences was then combined with data about health outcomes. Health outcomes data were based on the probabilities of mortality, morbidity (quality of life as represented by the presence or absence of symptoms and functional impairment) and return to former health state. The data were provided by Oregon's health service providers and by literature reviews, as in the earlier analysis. Health professionals were allowed to provide up to three outcome scenarios in addition to death and return to former health state.[12]

Having obtained a value for the net benefit of each procedure and ranked the condition/treatment pairs within categories according to this net benefit, the Commission then applied their "professional judgements and their interpretation of the community values to re-rate out-of-position items on the draft list" (Oregon Health Services Commission,[12] p.28). The final priority list, therefore, is to a large extent composed according to the value judgements of the members of the Health Services Commission. One member of the commission stated that "our own values and judgements. . . prevailed. . . where we felt that the other methods fell short" (Castanares in Fox and Leichter,[4] p.22), with a further member of the commission confirming the view that the list was the product of intense negotiation among members.[4] Cost became a consideration only when the Commissioners questioned the ranking of an item, or when two items were ranked equally according to the net benefit formula.[21]

The second version of the list was produced on 20 February 1991.[22] This list contained 709 condition/treatment pairs. The top 10 conditions and the bottom 10 conditions are shown in Table 2.2. The State of Oregon decided to fund the first 587 items on the priority list.[23] (Given the stated objective of covering most of the "very important" services, one critic has questioned whether funding up to line 650 would not be more appropriate.[24]) The proposed programme was estimated to cost at least 25% more than the current programme at that time.[25] Estimates of projected annual costs for varying levels of coverage were also produced.[26] If the Commission were to cover lines 1–310 (almost all "essential services") the cost would be US$0.7 million. If almost all "essential services" and approximately half of "very important services" were covered (lines 1–475) the cost would be US$16.5 million. If almost all "essential services" and "very important services" (lines 1–640) were covered the cost would be US$31.2 million. The cost of covering all 709 items was estimated to be approximately US$40.1 million.[26]

Oregon applied for a waiver of Medicaid requirements, required before the plan could be implemented, from the United States Health Care Financing Administration (HCFA) in August 1991, hoping to implement the new programme in July 1992, initially for a five-year period.[24] The state was proposing to monitor the effects of the programme on access, utilisation, outcomes, health status and costs during this five-year demonstration.[11] The US Administration, however, decided on 3 August 1992 that the plan was unacceptable in its state at that time because it would discriminate against individuals with physical or mental disabilities.[27] The Administration had come under pressure from groups representing people with disabilities and "right to life" groups, who held the view that the Oregon plan would violate the Americans with Disabilities Act by devaluing life with disability and using this as a basis for making funding decisions.[27,28] To some extent, therefore, the US

Table 2.2   Top and bottom of the second Oregon list: the 10 highest priority conditions and the 10 lowest priority conditions

Line	Diagnoses	Treatment
1	Pneumococcal pneumonia, other bacterial pneumonia, bronchopneumonia, influenza with pneumonia	Medical therapy
2	Tuberculosis	Medical therapy
3	Peritonitis	Medical and surgical therapy
4	Foreign body in pharynx, larynx, bronchus and oesophagus	Removal of foreign body
5	Appendicitis	Appendicectomy
6	Ruptured intestine	Repair
7	Hernia with obstruction and/or gangrene	Repair
8	Croup syndrome, acute laryngotracheitis	Medical therapy, intubation, tracheotomy
9	Acute orbital cellulitis	Medical therapy
10	Ectopic pregnancy	Surgery
700	Gynaecomastia	Mastopexy
701	Cyst of kidney, acquired	Medical and surgical treatment
702	End-stage HIV disease	Medical therapy
703	Chronic pancreatitis	Surgical treatment
704	Superficial wounds without infection and contusions	Medical therapy
705	Constitutional aplastic anaemia	Medical therapy
706	Prolapsed urethral mucosa	Surgical treatment
707	Central retinal artery occlusion	Paracentesis of aqueous
708	Extremely low birth weight (under 500 g) and under 23-week gestation	Life support
709	Anencephalous and similar anomalies and reduction deformities of the brain	Life support

Administration rejected the incorporation of public preferences into the prioritisation process, although there was some feeling that the plan was blocked mainly for political reasons during an election year.[28]

At this time, the US Administration recommended that Oregon should submit a revised application in which community values were not used, and ranking of condition/treatment pairs was not based on the telephone survey.[28] In response to this the Commission removed references to "quality of life" and "ability to function", instead relating all estimates of treatment benefit to the ability of a treatment to prevent death.[29] Cost was used to order items where benefit, as measured by prevention of death, was tied. Any further ties were ordered alphabetically. As in the second list, judgement was applied where items were felt to be wrongly positioned.[29]

As a further condition for the waiver approval Oregon was required to develop a process for reviewing treatments that appear below the funding lines, but are deemed to be medically appropriate in particular cases.[29] There are now set procedures for review on two main bases. The first is whether the treatment is covered for another condition which the patient has. The second is whether treatment of a non-funded condition/treatment pair would result in the same outcome as a funded condition/treatment pair.[29]

Following these changes and the election of President Clinton to the White House the fortunes of the Oregon Plan have undergone a reversal, with approval of the plan being granted in March 1993.[29-31] The Oregon Health Plan began on 1 February 1994, with 565 out of the 696 condition/treatment pairs in the modified list being funded.[29]

THE SUCCESS OF THE OREGON PLAN

At a two-day meeting about the Oregon Basic Health Services Act at the Hastings Center in January 1991, concerns were expressed about the standards for appraising health policy experiments. In particular, it was felt that the criteria for judging whether the Oregon plan was a success or a failure were unclear.[26] In practice, many criticisms of the plan have implicitly used the "ideal" as a comparison. The criterion for judging the Oregon plan should, however, be whether it improves on what is currently happening.[11]

Both criticisms of, and support for, the Oregon plan have concentrated on particular aspects of the plan. These aspects have ranged from broad questions about the need for any rationing of health care, and thus the necessity for a plan such as that devised by Oregon, to particular problems concerning the detailed methodology used by Oregon. In addition, there have also been concerns about the plan's implementation that may affect its ultimate success in changing the health care system in the State of Oregon. The Oregon plan may also be judged to have "succeeded" or "failed" in the extent to which it has brought priority setting onto the health care agenda, and the extent to which both its concepts and methodology are being repeated elsewhere.

Rather than look in detail at the issue of success, this section aims to consider how the Oregon plan has shed light on each of the conflicts discussed in Chapter 1. The conflicts will be discussed in the same order as they appear in that chapter, looking first at the explicit rationing, then at technical rationing, and finally at the equity–efficiency conflict.

OREGON: FROM IMPLICIT TO EXPLICIT RATIONING?

Medicaid ostensibly provides health care to those who cannot afford private health insurance. In practice, though, a large number of those unable to purchase private health insurance are also ineligible for Medicaid because their poverty is insufficiently great. The rules by which Medicaid operates have not, generally, been acknowledged as a form of explicit rationing in the USA, although that is how they appear to many overseas commentators (see Chapter 1). Thus although care is undoubtedly denied under both systems, the Oregon plan suffered far more criticism on the basis that it would be "rationing" care than Medicaid had previously been subject to.

Evidence for the implicit nature of rationing via Medicaid is provided by the number of critics who have simultaneously disputed the need for priority setting and criticised the Oregon plan on the basis that it is introducing rationing.[22,32,33] These commentators believe that there are no grounds upon which to ration health care, instead offering the argument that the desired level of health care can be achieved by eliminating wastage from the present system.[32,33]

The fact that the introduction of the Oregon plan has been seen by many as a move towards explicit rationing is interesting. In practice, the plan is a move from the rationing of care on the basis of individuals covered to the rationing of care on the basis of procedures covered. In some ways, the new plan does not represent a great departure from the original system in that its background assumptions are similar: that not everybody is able to have everything that they either want or need, and that therefore some system of priorities must be set.[1] The Oregon plan aims to replace rationing to a particular subset of the population (those below 100% of the federal poverty line) according to inability to pay, with rationing to this same subset of the population according to some combination of the effectiveness of medical treatment combined with a view of the public value of intervention. The fact that some have recognised rationing as occurring under both systems[34] has increased the level of support for the plan.

It is questionable whether a plan such as that implemented in Oregon would have ever become operational in a country moving from the more usual system of implicit rationing to an explicit form of rationing. Other countries, such as the UK, have experienced similar debates about treatments for individuals[35,36] as the Coby Howard experience in Oregon,[5] but these have not resulted in the level of support for explicit rationing that has been seen in Oregon. Perhaps the "all or nothing" nature of the Medicaid form of rationing is more unacceptable as a baseline situation than the more usual forms of implicit rationing such as occur in the UK, resulting in a greater degree of support for the subsequent explicit plan than might be found elsewhere.

There has also been discussion of the type of implicit rationing currently seen in the UK as an alternative to explicit rationing of the Oregon type. Explicit rationing has been rejected in favour of implicit rationing by some.[37,38] Critics such as Victor Fuchs have argued that rationing of care already exists and should be more systematic, but that it should be carried out implicitly at the patient–physician level.[38] Explicit rationing means accepting that not everything can be done for all individuals,[24] whereas implicit rationing may mean that this issue can be avoided:

> The greatest source of anguish in the implementation of the plan will come in learning how to live with, and to rationalize, its failure to

cover some people whose condition will pull at our sympathies. (Callahan,[1] p.85)

The Oregon plan has built into it, however, elements of implicit rationing. Oregon's legislature has emphasised a strategy which aims to reduce some of the problems involved in implementing the plan, by combining the priority list with capitation.[39] Contracts have been made with physician care organisations (PCOs), which receive a single monthly payment for each beneficiary in the PCO, and then provide services based upon the priority list. The priority list will define the benefit package on which the capitated rate will be based. Physicians will be able to prescribe treatments outside the benefit package, but without receiving an increase in payment.[39]

TECHNICAL RATIONING: THE DIFFICULTIES EXPOSED

The Oregon plan comprises technical rationing in all its glory. Although the principles behind each of the lists were not clearly enunciated, the aim was undoubtedly to use appropriate technical methodologies to set priorities. As a by-product of setting priorities for Oregon, the plan has exposed some of the shortcomings of technical rationing. There are problems with adequately including all the potential different types of patient with their different illnesses and potentially different treatments in the plan. The poor quality data upon which much of the plan is based provide another area of concern. These problems are not isolated from each other, however, but provide yet another example of conflict in the complex arena of technical priority setting. This conflict is discussed below, as is the potential for its resolution through pluralistic bargaining.

Heterogeneity of Patients

The definition of condition/treatment pairs in both of Oregon's first two lists was heavily criticised. Although 1600 condition/treatment pairs were identified for the first list, some pairs were still defined too broadly.[25] With the 709 condition/treatment pairs in the second list the problem was even more acute. Criticisms concerned the small number of pairs used, and thus their insensitivity to the possible number of diagnoses that exist. This lack of sensitivity has led to criticism that Oregon's lists considered only the average patient in each category, and do not allow for individual patient variation and different severities of illness for those with the same diagnosis.[1,6,24,40–43]

Henry Aaron makes the point that there are more than 10 000 diagnoses in the *Dictionary of Medical Diagnoses*, each of which includes patients with varying prognoses: "therefore if one wants to combine diagnoses with a reasonably sensitive awareness of the variability of potential outcomes, one is not talking about 10,000 categories, but some multiple of 10,000s" (Aaron,[44] p.109). The small number of pairs used by Oregon means that it is not possible to distinguish many medically heterogeneous situations.[44] In addition, the condition/treatment pairs do not allow for differences in the medical care provided within each diagnostic category.[44]

The condition/treatment pairs are also criticised for the lack of attention paid to the presence of co-morbidity.[24,40] This may lead to non-treatment of conditions that may be trivial for the patient without co-existing illness, but are serious in those with co-existing illness. Alternatively, it may lead to therapies that are usually very beneficial being performed for those who have severe co-morbidity, when in this latter case treatment is unlikely to be beneficial.[24]

The nature of technical rationing is that the technique is applied comprehensively across the chosen sphere. These criticisms levelled at Oregon's attempt to cover the entire domain of health care show the complexity associated even with classifying patients. The heterogeneity of patients may prove to be a major obstacle to the success of technical rationing.

Quality of Data

The first two Oregon lists each required data on the outcome of procedures. The first list additionally required information about cost and the second list required further information about public values in order to develop the ranked categorisations. These data were required for each of the 1600 condition/treatment pairs on the first list and each of the 709 condition/treatment pairs on the second list. Many general criticisms of these data have been voiced, for example, Alan Maynard's reference to the list as a "crude guesstimate" created in a "data free environment" (Maynard,[45] p.28). Difficulties in obtaining cost and outcome information with any degree of accuracy have been suggested by many critics as a reason for the failure of the cost–utility approach used in the first list,[19,25,40,41,46] with similar criticisms of the quality of the outcome data used in the second version of the list.[6,40,45]

The benefits of most medical and surgical procedures are not well understood:[47] experts do not agree, and the competing opinions of physicians are seldom based on good clinical trials.[45] Many estimates of effectiveness were made entirely on the basis of clinician judgement, incorporating the possibility of clinicians overestimating the benefit received by patients, either naïvely, or to enhance their own specialties.[19] Inadequate differentiation of the duration of the benefit of different treatments was made.[25] The social values embodied in the outcome measures have also been questioned. There is some doubt about whether they were captured accurately, particularly with respect to life-saving treatments.[25]

The cost figures used in the calculation were based on ranges of costs rather than particular costs per treatment. In addition, so-called "without treatment costs", the costs associated with not treating the patient, were not incorporated into the cost–utility calculation, thus biasing results. Neither costs nor benefits were discounted.

The methods by which public valuations were obtained, and even their use in the model, have been criticised on a number of grounds. The ranking of social values according to their frequency of mention at public meetings does not generate a credible listing of the health care priorities of the public,[26] and the telephone survey was unrepresentative of the population affected by the priority-setting exercise in terms of its inclusion of a very small number of households below the poverty line (those most affected by the Oregon plan).

Much of the data used in the Oregon plan was poor, but it has been stressed by some onlookers that decisions will always be made with inadequate data, and that the establishment of priorities cannot await the appearance of perfect data.[48] There is a question as to whether, within their resource constraints, the Oregon Commission could perhaps have made greater use of available data, or alternatively have attempted more sophisticated data collection methods. There is also a question as to whether it is practical to attempt to collect the sort of rigid data required for technical priority setting for such a large number of condition/treatment pairs.

Conflict: Assuming Heterogeneity versus Quality Data

The above discussion indicates that, within any resource constraint, there may be a direct conflict for technical priority-setting schemes. This conflict is between the assumptions made about heterogeneity and the acquisition of good quality data. A reduction in the number of condition/treatment pairs, could be expected to improve data quality, but would assume increased homogeneity among patients. An increased number of condition/treatment pairs would assume greater heterogeneity between patients, but at the probable expense of a reduction in data quality.

The impossibility of having what might be considered to be an appropriate number of condition/treatment pairs because of the data requirements that would be involved, means that technical methodologies for priority setting are likely to be extremely inflexible. A trade-off between explicitness and flexibility is introduced.[49] Including elements of pluralistic bargaining in the process may be one means of introducing more flexibility.

Resolving the Conflicts: Elements of Pluralistic Bargaining in the Oregon Plan

The final stage of developing the second list comprised the movement of items around the list on the basis of the Commissioners' judgements. The aim of these alterations was to change the rating for out-of-position items on the list,[12] thus allowing for difficulties caused by poor quality data. Had these judgements been made explicitly and openly defended, they would have provided an element of pluralistic bargaining in the plan.

Criticism of this stage of the methodology, however, has been associated with the lack of explicitness about these judgements.

Some authors have criticised the final methodology used in the process as being "opaque",[42] or have likened it to a "black box".[50] It is not clear on what basis the Commissioners made their adjustments[51] or how much weight the Commissioners' own value judgements were given, compared with the more factual information obtained about health outcomes or community values.[42] Although this process has been criticised on the basis that the replication of the plan in another state would produce a completely different list, given the sensitivity of the ranking to the Commissioners' judgements,[1,50] this in itself is not a problem: it may be that in a different locality with different values a different list would be expected. The problem is that lack of explicitness about the judgements makes them difficult to challenge. Open discussion, on the other hand, would have brought pluralistic bargaining into the Oregon experiment and ultimately made the process more acceptable to many critics.

Elements of pluralistic bargaining are, however, built into the Oregon plan at a clinical level. A process for the review of items, below the cut-off point but medically appropriate for particular cases, has been developed, whereby treatment will be provided for a non-funded condition/treatment pair if it would result in the same outcome as for a funded condition/treatment pair.[29]

THE EQUITY–EFFICIENCY CONFLICT

> The lack of any clear community historical tradition or present consensus on the setting of priorities, and the lack of any established method of determining the comparative importance to individual welfare of different procedures, make it problematic to evaluate the plan's design. (Callahan,[1] p.84)

Evaluation of the plan is particularly difficult given the lack of clarity with which Oregon expressed the principles upon which their plan was based. In fact, it is even questionable whether the Commission thought explicitly in terms of basing the plan on particular principles. What Oregon did express clearly was the desire to improve coverage with the plan – an element which may reflect a desire for efficiency (maximising health benefit) or equity (some form of equality of care). In terms of increasing coverage they have been successful, with eligibility expanding by 120 000 to cover all those below federal poverty guidelines,[52] albeit with a limited package of care. Whether this change in provision has increased equity is an issue which has been hotly disputed. It has been stated that by taking care away from some individuals to provide for a greater number, the plan will place an additional burden on the original group. Typically, this group comprises poor women and children who are already disadvantaged, and so the plan has been considered inequitable and unfair.[53–55] Other critics of the Oregon plan have protested that the plan is inequitable because the Medicaid programme has not been fed in its entirety into the prioritisation process. In fact, the groups for whom rationing will take place constitute about 70% of all Medicaid recipients but presently use only approximately 30% of the budget[22] and it has been said that these groups will therefore face an unfair burden.

Opponents of such views have, however, retorted that the present system is equally unfair. It has been said, in support of the Oregon plan, that there is great inequity in the present system, but that "blindness to this inequity is widespread among the critics of the Oregon plan" (Garland, Klevit and DiPrete,[10] p.308). The major concern must, therefore, be whether one system is preferable in some way (in terms of efficiency, equity or rights, for example) to the other. Some authors have concluded that the Oregon plan is more equitable than/an improvement over the present Medicaid system by comparing the benefits and coverage under each plan,[11,23] although others have been unable to make a judgement.[40]

The Plan: Equity or Efficiency?

How about the plan itself? What principles did it incorporate? In the first list the main principle used was almost certainly that of efficiency, that is, the maximisation of the benefit provided, in terms of perceived health gain, per unit of cost. Although this is not explicitly stated, the use of cost–utility analysis as a methodology implies efficiency as a basis for the priorities set. The first list produced by the Commission, however, appeared counterintuitive to Commissioners and provoked a high level of public criticism.[51,56] It was immediately decided that alternative methodologies should be considered. This has been interpreted by some as the failure of the principle of cost–utility analysis.[17]

It is interesting to question what is meant by the "counterintuitive" ordering of condition/treatment pairs. Although there are problems familiar to all technical methods concerning the inadequacies of data used in the analysis and the problems in defining sufficiently well the condition/treatment pairs, there is a more important issue to consider. The ordering of a list based on an efficiency principle is based on both the benefit obtained from a treatment and the cost of that treatment. At the top of the list there will not only be those treatments which provide much benefit. There may also be treatments which provide some benefit but at a very low cost. Intuition though might suggest that the most beneficial treatments appear at the top of the list. After all, intuitively it appears to be wrong to state that treatment of, say, ingrowing toe-nails should have higher priority than treatment of appendicitis. Thus, the inconsistencies in the list criticised by some observers may not in fact be inconsistencies – rather it may be the intuitive interpretation that causes apparent inconsistencies.[57] As David Eddy explains: ". . . it is important to understand that a priority-setting process based on cost–utility ratios should not be expected to rank services according to our intuitive sense of their 'importance' or degree of benefit. . . If you want to check the results against your intuition, you should compare the volumes of different services that can be offered with a particular amount of resources. . . The intuition to compare adjacent services directly (one to one) is not only inappropriate, it is misleading."[57]

It cannot, therefore, be claimed that efficiency as a principle upon which to base priority setting failed in the Oregon experiment. Rather it was the expectation that the set of priorities produced on this basis should look "intuitive" that was wrong. The failure of the Commission and many onlookers both to comprehend and accept the nature of the resulting list is, however, more of a concern. If the only people to whom such a list looks acceptable are economists, setting priorities based on efficiency is unlikely to be successful. Interestingly, however, there have been criticisms of the methodology used for the second list for making no use of information about costs![50]

The second list produced by the Oregon Commission was perceived as being more intuitively correct by observers of the Commission's work, and therefore provoked less of an outburst. The principle upon which the second list is based, however, is much less clear (Broome has stated that he found "the criteria used as clear as mud"! (Broome,[58] p.355)), but there are strong indications that the list is based on the equity principle of equal treatment for equal need, where need is defined as ability to benefit. The "rule of rescue"[17] is embraced in this list, and the more intuitively correct ordering achieved also provides evidence that need was the overriding basis of the second list. Use of this principle implies that there are some health needs that are so important that they must always be met before other health needs are considered. Such a proposition is supported by some (for example, Hadorn feels that the "rule of rescue" is so important that it always outweighs other considerations[17]), but questioned by many others.[1,50]

Discrimination in the Oregon Plan

The second list produced by Oregon was refused a federal waiver on the basis that it contravened the Americans with Disabilities Act implemented in July 1992.[27,28] It was felt that the weights obtained through the telephone survey were equivalent to the value placed on a person's life, and it was also considered possible to equate symptom descriptions in this score with definitions of disabilities. Thus the community values used in the ranking of condition/treatment pairs were guilty of discriminating against the disabled. This has been disputed in a number of academic papers. Broome states that the plan was not guilty in this way – although it would have been if it had been consistent in the aim of using resources to do the most good.[59] He states that because the plan ranked only condition/treatment pairs, as opposed to treatments for individuals, it could not discriminate against any particular individuals, except if particular diseases also discriminate in whom they affect.[58,59]

Kaplan also disagreed that the plan was discriminatory.[60] He showed that preferences did not differ greatly across social or demographic groups. In particular he compared ratings of those Oregon citizens who had been in a wheelchair with the preferences of those who had not had such an experience and found that there was little difference[60] – of course, what is meant by "have been in a wheelchair" is unclear. Kaplan also states that any bias that does exist is in favour of those with disabilities, because they will have a lower initial health score which can be improved by a greater amount.[60]

CONCLUSION: THE IMPLICATIONS FROM OREGON

Many issues have been highlighted by Oregon's experience, and one conclusion drawn by many onlookers so far, is that the experiment has shown that there is no quick or easy technological fix to the question of setting priorities.[61,62] The Oregon plan has made quite obvious many of the limitations of technical methods for explicit priority setting.

Oregon has been particularly successful in bringing priority setting onto the agenda for health care. The volume of work that has been produced both in support of, and opposition to, the Oregon plan shows the extent to which priority setting in health care is now considered to be an important topic. The potential for using similar plans has also met with a considerable amount of interest both in the United States and in other countries grappling with the problems of rising health care costs. Attempts have been made to replicate the Oregon exercise in some district health authorities in the UK,[63–65] and suggestions have also been made that the approach should be investigated with respect to its usefulness in Australia.[7]

One example of an attempt to base priority setting in the UK on the Oregon experiment, is that of the Mid Essex health authority.[64,65] Here selective use has been made of specific tools used in Oregon, rather than an attempt to import the approach in its entirety.[65] This health authority initiated a series of fora attended by representatives of the health authority, members of voluntary organisations, and the community health council. During these fora an introduction was given about the need for the public to be involved in assessing health priorities, a video of the Oregon experiment was shown, and participants were asked to complete the Oregon questionnaires. The questionnaires were completed individually in the first instance, and small groups then attempted to reach a consensus. The results indicated that individuals held many similar values, attitudes and beliefs about health care.[64] In addition to the use of the Oregon tools, participants were also asked to rank a number of treatments for various conditions based on a questionnaire developed by the TV programme "Public Eye". The orderings provided by the public and by clinicians were similar, with hip replacements, cataract removal and heart bypass surgery heading the list, and treatment for advanced Parkinson's disease, treatment for advanced lung cancer, and heart and liver transplants coming at the bottom of the list.[64] Wandsworth health authority has also planned to use Oregon's category rating method as a means of setting priorities, although concern about how the public may react has slowed the exercise.[65]

The contribution of the Oregon plan may thus be less for the details of the plan itself than in its exploration of the concept of technical rationing. Both the plan itself, and the critical assessment which has followed it, have raised many previously hidden issues. Although the state of Oregon had the objective of setting priorities in order to increase the coverage of the population, it had no clear idea about the ways in which this should be achieved. The development of the plan was characterised by repeated reaction to events beyond the Commissioners' control: the media and public outrage at the death of Coby Howard; the "unintuitive" ordering of the first list of priorities; the refusal by the Federal Government to grant a waiver for the second plan. The Oregon plan thus exposed a previously neglected aspect of technical rationing: that it may produce results which are unexpected and/or unacceptable to some. With technical models the nature of the priorities that will be set are not discussed prior to the formation of a list, and so the production of the list will almost inevitably cause debate, some of which may be unfavourable. This contrasts with the more open nature of pluralistic bargaining, in which a wide range of issues are inevitably discussed as part of the process by which priorities are set.

Finally, it is questionable whether the Oregon plan has reduced or increased the confusion that surrounds the whole area of priority setting. Limited attempts to repeat the plan have not followed it in its entirety, but have selected particular aspects. This is principally because the Oregon experiment is not one plan, but represents several attempts to set acceptable priorities within the technical tradition. Those involved in the Oregon plan, have themselves stated that the approach should be seen, not as offering a final solution, but as a dynamic process.[66] Ultimately, Oregon has shown that a purist technical approach to setting priorities cannot be imposed on a health system. Public and professional reactions at each stage have led, unintentionally, to Oregon's technical plan becoming in part an exercise in priority setting via the political process.

REFERENCES

1. Callahan D. Ethics and priority setting in Oregon. *Health Affairs* 1991; **Summer**: 78–87.
2. Crawshaw R, Garland M, Hines B, Anderson B. Developing principles for prudent health care allocation. The continuing Oregon experiment. *Western J Med* 1990; **152**(4): 441–6.
3. Welch HG, Larson EB. Dealing with limited resources. The Oregon decision to curtail funding for organ transplantation. *N Engl J Med* 1988; **319**(3): 171–3.
4. Fox DM, Leichter HM. Rationing care in Oregon: the new accountability. *Health Affairs* 1991; **Summer**: 7–27.
5. Klevit HD, Bates AC, Castanares T, Kirk EP, Sipes-Metzler PR, Wopat R. Prioritization of health care services. A progress report by the Oregon Health Services Commission. *Arch Intern Med* 1991; **151**: 912–16.
6. Honigsbaum F. *Who shall live? Who shall die? – Oregon's health financing proposals*. King's Fund College, London, 1991.
7. Street A, Richardson J. The value of health care: what can we learn from Oregon? *Aust Health Review* 1992; **15**(2): 124–34.
8. Goldsmith MF. Oregon pioneers 'more ethical' Medicaid coverage with priority-setting project. *J Am Med Assoc* 1989; **262**(2):176–7.
9. McBride G. Oregon revises health care priorities. *BMJ* 1991; **302**: 549.
10. Garland M, Klevit H, DiPrete B. Policy analysis or polemic on Oregon's rationing plan? [letter]. *Health Affairs* 1991; **Winter**: 307–10.
11. Eddy DM. Oregon's plan. Should it be approved? *J Am Med Assoc* 1991; **266**(17): 2439–45.
12. Oregon Health Services Commission. *Prioritization of Health Services. A report to the Governor and Legislature*. Oregon Health Services Commission, 1991.

13. Drummond MF, Stoddart GL, Torrance GW. *Methods for the economic evaluation of health care programmes.* Oxford University Press, Oxford, 1987.
14. Kaplan RM, Anderson JP. The General Health Policy Model: an integrated approach. In: Spilker B, ed. *Quality of life assessments in clinical trials.* Raven Press, New York, 1990: 131–49.
15. Kaplan RM, Bush JW. Health-related quality of life measurement for evaluation research and policy analysis. *Health Psychol* 1981; **1**: 61–80.
16. Morell V. Oregon puts bold health plan on ice. *Science* 1990; **249**: 468–71.
17. Hadorn DC. Setting health care priorities in Oregon. Cost-effectiveness meets the rule of rescue. *J Am Med Assoc* 1991; **265**(17): 2218–25.
18. Buist A. *The Oregon experiment: combining expert opinion and community values to set health care priorities.* Health Economics Research Group, Brunel University, 1992.
19. Kaplan RM. A quality-of-life approach to health resource allocation. In: Strosberg MA, Weiner JM, Baker R, Fein A, eds. *Rationing America's medical care: the Oregon plan and beyond.* The Brookings Institution, Washington, DC, 1992: 60–77.
20. Morell V. Listing to starboard: the Oregon formula. *Science* 1990; **249**: 470.
21. Garland MJ. Rationing in public: Oregon's priority setting methodology. In: Strosberg MA, Weiner JM, Baker R, Fein IA, eds. *Rationing America's medical care: the Oregon plan and beyond.* The Brookings Institution, Washington, DC, 1992: 37–59.
22. Brown LD. The national politics of Oregon's rationing plan. *Health Affairs* 1991; **Summer**: 28–51.
23. Robinson EL. The Oregon Basic Health Services Act – a model for state reform. *Vanderbilt Law Review* 1992; **45**(4): 977–1014.
24. Steinbrook R, Lo B. The Oregon Medicaid demonstration project – will it provide adequate medical care? *N Engl J Med* 1992; **326**(5): 340–4.
25. Eddy DM. What's going on in Oregon? *J Am Med Assoc* 1991; **266**(3): 417–20.
26. Dougherty CJ. Setting health care priorities. Oregon's next steps. *Hastings Center Report* 1991; **May–June**: 1–9.
27. Dixon J. Approval denied for Oregon experience. *Lancet* 1992; **340**: 418–19.
28. McBride G. Bush vetoes health care rationing in Oregon. *BMJ* 1992; **305**: 437–8.
29. Sipes-Metzler PR. Oregon health plan: ration or reason. *J Med Philos* 1994; **19**: 305–14.
30. Roberts J. Clinton gives go ahead to Oregon's health plan. *BMJ* 1993; **306**: 811.

31. McCarthy M. Clinton approval for Oregon health "rationing" plan. *Lancet* 1993; **341**: 817.
32. Sanders B. A national health care alternative to the Oregon plan. In: Strosberg MA, Weiner JM, Baker R, Fein IA, eds. *Rationing America's medical care: the Oregon plan and beyond*. The Brookings Institution, Washington, DC, 1992: 119–22.
33. Tartaglia AP. Is talk of rationing premature? In: Strosberg MA, Weiner JM, Baker R, Fein IA, eds. *Rationing America's medical care: the Oregon plan and beyond*. The Brookings Institution, Washington, DC, 1992: 144–50.
34. Callahan D. Evaluating the Oregon priority plan. *J Am Geriatr Soc* 1991; **39**: 622–3.
35. Anon. Who should live, who should die? *Which* 1994; **July**: 50–3.
36. Hall C, Mackinnon I. Cancer girl loses fight for treatment. *The Independent* 1995; **11 March**: 1.
37. Ayres SM. Rationality, not rationing, in health care. In: Strosberg MA, Weiner JM, Baker R, Fein IA, eds. *Rationing America's medical care: the Oregon plan and beyond*. The Brookings Institution, Washington, DC, 1992: 132–43.
38. Dixon J, Welch HG. Priority setting: lessons from Oregon. Lancet 1991; **337**: 891–4.
39. Welch HG, Fisher ES. Oregon's priority list – pertinence to radiologists. *Invest Radiol* 1992; **27**(5): 379–84.
40. Nelson RM, Drought T. Justice and the moral acceptability of rationing medical care: the Oregon experiment. *J Med Philos* 1992; **17**: 97–117.
41. Bowling A. Setting priorities in health: the Oregon experiment (part 2). *Nursing Standard* 1992; **6**(38): 28–30.
42. Klein R. Warning signals from Oregon. The different dimensions of rationing need untangling. *BMJ* 1992; **304**: 1457–8.
43. Relman AS. Assessing the Oregon plan. [letter]. *Issues Sci Technol* 1991; **Summer**: 14–15.
44. Aaron HJ. The Oregon experiment. In: Strosberg MA, Weiner JM, Baker R, Fein IA, eds. *Rationing America's medical care: the Oregon plan and beyond*. The Brookings Institution, Washington, DC, 1992: 107–11.
45. Maynard A. On the Oregon trail. *Health Service J* 1991; **23 May**: 28.
46. McBride G. Rationing health care in Oregon. *BMJ* 1990; **301**: 355–6.
47. Langfitt TW. Assessing the Oregon plan. *Issues Sci Technol* 1991; **Summer**: 15–16.
48. Welch HG. Health care tickets for the uninsured. First class, coach or standby? *N Engl J Med* 1989; **321**(18): 1261–4.
49. Lansdown R. Oregon health decisions: common sense pursued. *J R Soc Med* 1992; **85**: 501–2.

50. Granneman TW. Priority setting: A sensible approach to Medicaid policy? *Inquiry* 1991; **28**: 300–5.
51. Daniels N. Justice and health care rationing: lessons from Oregon. In: Strosberg MA, Weiner JM, Baker R, Fein IA, eds. *Rationing America's medical care: the Oregon plan and beyond.* The Brookings Institution, Washington, DC, 1992: 185–95.
52. Department of Human Resources, Office of Medical Assistance Programs. *The Oregon Health Plan.* Department of Human Resources, Portland, 1994.
53. Rosenbaum S. Poor women, poor children, poor policy: the Oregon Medicaid experiment. In: Strosberg MA, Weiner JM, Baker R, Fein IA, eds. *Rationing America's medical care: the Oregon plan and beyond.* The Brookings Institution, Washington, DC, 1992: 91–106.
54. Garland MJ, Hasnain R. Health care in common: setting priorities in Oregon. *Hastings Center Report* 1990; **Sept/Oct**: 16–18.
55. Rosenbaum S. Mothers and children last: the Oregon Medicaid experiment. *Am J Law Med* 1992; **18**(1–2): 97–126.
56. Strosberg MA. Introduction. In: Strosberg MA, Wiener JM, Baker R, Fein IA, eds. *Rationing America's medical care: the Oregon plan and beyond.* The Brookings Institution, Washington, DC, 1992: 3–11.
57. Eddy DM. Oregon's methods. Did cost-effectiveness analysis fail? *J Am Med Assoc* 1991; **266**(15): 2135–41.
58. Broome J. 'Rationing America's Medical Care: The Oregon Plan and Beyond' edited by Martin A Strosberg, Joshua M Wiener, Robert Baker and I Alan Fein. The Brookings Institution, 1992. [review]. *Bioethics* 1993; **7**: 351–8.
59. Broome J. Fairness versus doing the most good. *Hastings Center Report* 1994; **July–August**: 36–9.
60. Kaplan RM. Application of a general health policy model in the American health care crisis. *J R Soc Med* 1993; **86**: 277–81.
61. Klein R. On the Oregon trail: rationing health care. *BMJ* 1991; **302**: 1–2.
62. May A. Perfect purchasing. *Health Service J* 1992; **16 July**: 23–4.
63. Geller RJ. Personal communication, 1992.
64. Bowling A. Setting priorities in health: the Oregon experiment (part 1). *Nursing Standard* 1992; **6**(37): 29–32.
65. Ham C, Honigsbaum F, Thompson D. *Priority Setting for Health Gain.* Department of Health, London, 1993.
66. Crawshaw R. The Oregon Medicaid controversy. *N Engl J Med* 1992; **327**: 642.

CHAPTER THREE

JOANNA COAST

Core Services: Pluralistic Bargaining in New Zealand

Oregon does not provide the only international experience from which to learn. In separate attempts to decide on the basic, or core, services that should be provided by the health care system free of charge, whole nations are also grappling with these problems. New Zealand is one of these nations, and this chapter will concentrate upon its experience of defining *core services*. The experience of New Zealand was chosen as a contrast to that of Oregon because of its quite deliberate choice to reject technical methods of priority setting and instead to take a different approach. This approach is characterised by its emphasis on consensus, and its similarity to the ideals of pluralistic bargaining as advocated by Klein.[1] Hence, examination of priority setting in New Zealand provides useful information about how such an approach might work in practice.

It is worth stating here, however, that other countries, such as Sweden, Norway and the Netherlands, are also attempting to define basic or core services.[2] For example, in the Netherlands a comprehensive report on priority setting, *Choices in Health Care*, was published in 1992 by the Government Committee on Choices in Health Care.[3] Whilst *Choices for Health Care* makes a number of recommendations regarding how choices should be made, there has been no attempt, however, to put the report into practice. Although the approach is not discussed in detail here, there are parallels

Priority Setting: The Health Care Debate.
Edited by J. Coast, J. Donovan and S. Frankel.   © 1996 John Wiley & Sons Ltd.

between this approach and that taken in New Zealand which will be mentioned throughout the chapter.

The work on priority setting in New Zealand began in 1991, but has not generated anything like the level of intellectual comment resulting from the Oregon plan. Indeed, its efforts have, to date, made relatively little impact on discussions about priority setting, although the route it has taken towards setting core services has been dramatically different from the route taken by Oregon and may be much more useful to many countries aiming to move from implicit towards explicit rationing.

The chapter begins by detailing the work carried out in New Zealand by the Core Services Committee. The contribution of these efforts to understanding the conflicts described in Chapter 1 will then be discussed.

CORE SERVICES: THE BEST OF HEALTH

The New Zealand Department of Health has been tackling the problem of priority setting – or deciding on "core services" – since the early 1990s. The New Zealand statement of health policy *Your Health and the Public Health*, otherwise known as the "Green and White Paper", stated that, as part of the major reform of the New Zealand health system, the government would explicitly define core health services.[4] A consultation document detailing various options was therefore sent out in November 1991 with a request for responses by early January 1992.[5] There were two broad options for setting core services discussed in this document.[5] The first was the option of a detailed priority-ranked list with highly centralised decision-making. The Oregon experiment was given as an example of such a list. The second option was described as a "general" list which would specify core services in terms of broad categories of health service while leaving more detailed decisions about specific priorities to different local levels and thus allowing for regional variations and greater individual choice by clinicians and patients.[5]

Submissions resulting from this document were published in May 1992.[4] A total of 1586 submissions were received in response to the first Core Services document. Approximately 1250 of these commented on the definition of core health services, with around 700 making substantive comment. A total of 821 organisations are listed as having commented on the issue of core services, including area health boards, local government, voluntary agencies, public agencies, community-based health groups, women's, Maori, Pacific Island and church groups and school boards of trustees.[4] Submissions are concentrated among groups with some relationship to health care, either through professional organisations, local health groups or voluntary organisations.

The foreword to the *Review of Submissions* stated that:

> The clear preference is for a general positive list, allowing for regional prioritisation, coupled with a short negative listing of those services to be excluded from public funding (The Bridgeport Group,[4] p.v).

The need for flexibility in priority setting was noted, both in terms of the need for clinical decisions to reflect the needs of individual patients and the need for culturally appropriate core health services.[4] In addition to the discussion of the options as laid out in the original document, a number of other themes were identified in the submissions. The most consistent commitment was to a scheme with universal access, with provision of health services for those in need, regardless of financial or other circumstances, being seen as essential.[4] The necessity for a framework of moral and ethical values upon which to base core services was also discussed. The recommendation that this framework should be developed with full consultation is a reflection of the more general desire among respondents for continuing consultation.[4] It is interesting to note from the submissions that there was little support for expenditure control as an objective for the health care system.[4]

The submissions also contained some concerns about the whole policy of setting core services.[4] A number of submissions questioned whether there was sufficient available information in New Zealand about benefits of treatments, cost of treatments and the health status of the community from which to make informed and sound decisions. Others questioned whether the benefits of the approach of defining "core services" were justified by the costs. Concern was also expressed that defining core services may have undesirable effects in discriminating against certain groups of people such as low-income women and their dependants.[4]

In March 1992, while these submissions were still being analysed, a National Advisory Committee on Core Health and Disability Support Services was set up with the task of advising the Government on the health and disability support services that the Government should purchase.[6] In essence the role of this committee is to determine how priorities should be set and what those priorities are. The work of the Committee has been characterised by a number of approaches, many relating to the submissions contained in the report by the Bridgeport group.[4] At all levels public consultation has been extensive, including ethics forums for the public,[7] public forums,[8–10] public meetings including *hui*,[6,11,12] consensus conferences with lay participation,[6,11–13] a questionnaire for the public[14] and public documents with the aim of acquiring information about public views on priority setting, sent out for consultation purposes.[14,15]

The remainder of this section will discuss in detail the parallel approaches followed by the Committee.

A GENERAL LIST APPROACH

The Core Services Committee has chosen explicitly not to pursue the option of a detailed list of priorities such as that developed by Oregon. Such a policy was rejected on the basis that it would be impossible to implement: either it would have to be very broad and thus meaningless, or it would have to be very rigid and therefore inevitably inflexible and unfair.[16,17] Further, it is stated that such lists are unable to tailor services to the needs of individuals and communities.[12] In essence this forms a rejection of technical priority-setting methods.

Instead the Core Services Committee has chosen to identify broad areas of priorities: the general list approach described in the initial consultation document.[5] The working assumption of the Committee has been that current service provision comprises the core, but that, gradually over time, this core will change to reflect the priorities determined by the Committee.[6,11,12]

Initially the Committee aimed to combine the general list with a short list of exclusions, with the Committee reporting in 1992 that it had had "initial thoughts on which services may be of lesser priority" (Core Services Committee,[6] 1992, p.8). Through public consultation, lower priority had tentatively been accorded to: maintaining life at any cost; unnecessary "high tech" intervention; surgical procedures that benefit relatively few people; and technology/pharmaceuticals whose cost-effectiveness has not been demonstrated.[6] Some specific suggestions for limits had included limiting transplant surgery, cosmetic surgery, genetics, fertility services, brain surgery and treatment of sports injuries and intensive care at the beginning and end of life.[6] The report published at the end of 1994, however, abandoned the idea of negative lists or service exclusions on the basis that they would be arbitrary and unsustainable. It was also stated, however, that services that would not generally be included in the core would include experimental technologies, services without any demonstrated effectiveness and conditions where treatment does not usually rank as a high priority.[12] Rather than identifying whole services which will or will not be provided, the aim has been to describe the circumstances in which access will be provided to publicly funded services.[12]

The first report of the Core Services Committee published in November 1992 provided a "stocktake", looking in detail at the current provision of health services in New Zealand.[6] More importantly, it also set out the different ways in which priorities would be considered at different levels. Specifically, priority setting in New Zealand has been divided into two levels: setting priorities between services and setting priorities within services.

PUBLIC MEETINGS AND PRIORITIES BETWEEN SERVICES

At the level of setting priorities between services, the committee appears to have concentrated heavily on its consultations with the public. Three broad priorities identified from consultation with the public in September and October 1992 were recommended in the first report: mental health and substance abuse services, children's health services and integrated community care services.[6] Three supplementary priorities were also noted: emergency ambulance services, hospice services, habilitation/rehabilitation services. These six areas were reconfirmed as priorities in the following year's report, following a total of 19 public meetings at which the priorities were confirmed, with the recommendations that they should be given progressively more emphasis.[11] In the 1994 report, although it was stated that the three priority areas were reconfirmed, the titles had been shortened and altered slightly.[12] In particular, the third priority had been renamed – from "integrated community care services, including appropriate and culturally acceptable services for Maori" to "Maori health".[12] This is not highlighted as a change in priorities, but differences in the annual report imply a strong change in emphasis – although nowhere is it stated that the priorities are anything other than "confirmed"![12] It is interesting to speculate as to how and why this evidently political decision came about, and what this means for public consultation at this level.

In the public meetings held during 1993 at which these priorities had been confirmed, the Committee was also urged "to make sure priorities translate into service delivery" (Core Services Committee,[11] 1993, p.30). In that report the Committee stated that in the future they would report on the purchasing decisions made by Regional Health Authorities to meet the priorities identified by New Zealanders.[11] In the third report in November 1994 the Committee attempted to do this.[12] For example, in the area of mental health it noted the progress that had been made: the Minister of Health had directed the development of a comprehensive mental health strategy; the Government had commissioned a "stocktake" in late 1993; and the Government had instructed that specific levels of services should be set for mental health services.[12] Some of these had already been set at the time of this report, while others were in the process of development.[12]

CONSENSUS CONFERENCES AND PRIORITIES WITHIN SERVICES

At the level of setting priorities within services, the Committee has chosen the route of consensus conferences to provide recommendations on how equity of access and better outcomes for patients could be addressed.[6] The Committee has chosen to begin the process of defining core services by looking at those high-cost and high-volume services which, the Committee states, offer the most potential for improvement and for redirecting resources.[12]

Consensus conferences have been attended by both health professionals and expert lay people such as patients with the relevant condition or representatives of voluntary groups. The recommendations resulting from the conferences have taken the form of "boundary guidelines".[6] These guidelines are intended to apply in usual circumstances in the chosen areas of clinical practice, but it has been explicitly stated that in unusual circumstances clinical discretion is important and guidelines may be of less value.[6] The guidelines are intended not only to offer guidance to purchasers and providers, but also to help inform the public of the circumstances when services are likely to be publicly funded.[12] By 1994 the Committee's message relating to guidelines had become more strongly related to issues of cost-effectiveness, with statements that some of the guidelines would "offer significant and clinically justifiable resource savings" (Core Services Committee,[12] p.37) and thus could be used to maximise benefit for the available resources. There is also, in this report, explicit acknowledgement that these guidelines may not opt for technically superior treatments where other approaches are more cost-effective.[12]

In the first report boundary guidelines were provided for nine clinical areas, including major joint replacement, coronary artery bypass grafting and angioplasty; management of end-stage kidney failure, aftercare of normal deliveries and prescribing minor tranquillisers.[6] In the report at the end of 1993 the recommendations from these nine conferences as well as a further two were confirmed following circulation for wider consultation with sector professionals and community experts.[11] Further consensus conferences were also held during that year and the next, in areas such as hormone replacement therapy, alcohol and drug problems and the management of dyspepsia.[11,12]

Attempts have also been made, using consensus approaches, to look at both broader and more detailed issues. Four broad issues concerning access to services were identified from the detailed consensus conferences described above, and in 1993 the Core Services Committee published *Seeking Consensus,* a document asking for feedback and suggestions from the public in these areas.[13] The four areas identified were: the management of waiting lists; local, regional and national services; primary medical care; and health and disability support service planning.[13]

In 1994 the Committee piloted a new consultation initiative, involving panel discussions between randomly recruited members of the general public and health professionals over whether, and if so which, social factors should be taken into account when selecting people for surgery.[10,12] These forums related specifically to the development of priority criteria for cataract surgery, and coronary artery bypass graft and angioplasty. The criteria comprise both clinical and social factors, and the aim of the public forums was to consult over the social factors. The resultant criteria for cataract surgery contain clinical factors reflecting visual acuity, glare and other visual defects, and social factors reflecting limitations on activities, the need to work or provide care for dependants, the need to drive, and the extent of other disabilities.[12] For coronary revascularisation, prognostic factors comprise 90% of the priority score and social factors the remaining 10%.[12]

A MORAL AND ETHICAL FRAMEWORK

The second report of the Core Services Committee in 1993 tentatively outlined four broad principles on which the public funding of health services should be based.[11] These four basic principles were that the treatment or service:

- provides *benefit;*
- is *value for money;*
- is a *fair* use of public money;
- is consistent with *communities' values.*

The principles are founded on the idea of what is referred to as an "individual benefit" criterion for deciding on future core services, with the concern being whether a particular service should be funded for a particular person at a particular time.[12]

Public consultation about this framework took place during 1993/94 with the publication of *The best of health 2: How we decide on the health and disability support services we value most*.[12,15] In addition to outlining and explaining this framework, *The best of health 2* reiterates the need to make choices about health care and describes other approaches to priority setting such as the Oregon experiment and the use of QALYs.[15] Submissions in response to this document as well as other comments made at meetings were felt to support these principles and the Committee concluded that it was an appropriate framework within which to advise on the relative priorities of publicly funded services.[12]

THE SUCCESS OF *CORE SERVICES*

Up to 1995, then, it appears that New Zealand had made considerable progress in developing its priorities. As with the Oregon Plan, judging the success or otherwise of the *Core Services* approach is very difficult. Again, therefore, as in the preceding chapter on Oregon, this section considers the lessons provided by the *Core Services* approach for each of the conflicts discussed in Chapter 1. The conflicts will be discussed in the same order as they appear in that chapter, looking first at the issue of explicit rationing, then at pluralistic bargaining as the basis for developing priorities and at the form that lay participation has taken in New Zealand. The final section looks at those elements of technical priority setting which are also evident in the *Core Services* approach.

FROM IMPLICIT TO EXPLICIT RATIONING?

Prior to the creation of the Core Services Committee in New Zealand there were already limits to the care that was publicly funded. As the earlier documents produced by the Ministry of Health state, some services were, by implication, in the "core" and others were not.[5] Services that were not publicly funded in 1991 when the Committee was set up included most adult dental work, liposuction, chiropody and optometry.[5] There were also other services, such as liver transplantation (provided overseas), upon which limits were set.[5] Apart from these few, relatively explicit, exclusions, however, the majority of care in New Zealand was rationed implicitly in a manner similar to that in the UK: with a fixed sum of money provided to each health board and decisions about the provision of specific forms of care for specific patients left to individual clinicians.

To what extent has this changed? In its first three years, the Core Services Committee has regularly and emphatically rejected the notion of a detailed priority list in an Oregon-type format. Recommendations have stated that the broad range of current provision should act as a baseline for core services and that this pattern of services should gradually shift over time through the implementation of the priorities.[6] So is this still implicit rationing?

As with all attempts at setting priorities the degree to which priority setting can become explicit is limited. As the early Core Services documentation states:

> It is worth noting that no list could ever be so detailed that all variations and individual circumstances were taken account of, thus removing the need for some decision-making at the doctor–patient level. (Minister of Health,[5] p.8).

In New Zealand the setting of priorities is now an acknowledged aspect of health care provision, and as the Committee themselves state, they have tried to ensure that the process for defining which services should be publicly funded "is conducted in a more open and nationally agreed way, rather than in the former sometimes random way which took place generally behind closed doors" (Core Services Committee,[11] p.42). The process of priority setting has certainly become more explicit as a result of the determination to set core services, although the route taken is a much more gradual one than that of the Oregon plan. Rather than adopting a technical rationing scheme, the Committee has taken the route of pluralistic bargaining. The specific form that this has taken is discussed below.

GETTING THE PROCESS RIGHT: PLURALISTIC BARGAINING IN NEW ZEALAND

The technical rationing approach of a detailed list based upon a specific methodology has been rejected by the New Zealand Core Services Committee. Initial consultation showed a widespread preference for an approach that would combine a broad and general set of priorities with the flexibility to allow for some regional variation and prioritisation.[4] A "general list" of this type was advanced by respondents on the bases that it would be more widely understood, more amenable to community participation, less open to capture by stronger interest groups and allow more scope for independent clinical judgement.[4] Flexibility was felt to be important because each region has unique health requirements, because there are different cultural requirements for health care and because rural areas have different requirements from urban areas.[4] There was little support for detailed ranking of priorities for administrative, medical and ethical reasons. Such a list was felt to be too complex, time-consuming and costly, and likely to result in both practical problems of implementation for clinicians, and moral problems of discrimination.[4] The Committee has stood by these views, stating that detailed lists are both overly simplistic and potentially unfair. Their alternative approach to core services is one of whether and when a service should be publicly funded.[11]

The priority-setting process in New Zealand acknowledges that priority setting takes place at different levels. Although identifying six levels at which priorities are set (between health and other services, between regions, between services, between specialties, between treatments, and between individuals) two levels are approached explicitly: within services and between services.[6] At these different levels it is recognised that different types of decision are required, and that alternative approaches will reflect the most appropriate ways of making these decisions. Even for the "within services" approach of guidelines, however, it is explicitly accepted that different individuals may have different needs, and that professional judgement is needed to identify when the guidelines should be applied.[12] This implies acceptance that guidelines will not be comprehensive enough to cover all clinical eventualities.

At all levels the process is one of consensus. The aim has not been to set one overarching objective to be met by the health care system (as would be usual for technical methodologies), but instead to allow all those involved in setting priorities to bring their own objectives to the bargaining table. Through collective discussion, and eventual consensus, priorities can then be set.

The approach is undoubtedly one of incrementalism. It is accepted that defining core services is a dynamic process that will never be finished.[5] Presently funded services are seen as the core services, and changes to that core will be "well-researched and gradual" (Core Services Committee,[6] p.63). Because the process is so gradual there are not the problems of excessive data requirements that are faced by more technical rationing schemes. In choosing where to begin, however, the Committee has opted for those high-cost and high-volume procedures that affect greater numbers and offer most potential for increased benefit and the reallocation of resources.[12]

LAY PARTICIPATION IN SETTING CORE SERVICES

The whole approach to core services in New Zealand appears to place a heavy emphasis on involving a variety of individuals and groups in the process of priority setting. [This is paralleled by the approach recommended for the Netherlands by *Choices in Health Care*, where the Committee recommended that public discussion about choices in health care should be encouraged, and that patient/consumer organisations should contribute to both this discussion and discussion about the individual responsibilities of the insured.[3]] In the initial consultation document it was stated that "we need to strike a balance between public consultation, individual choice and expert input into the decision-making process" (Minister of Health,[5] p.4). Clearly, one reason for the extent of consultation is that there is unmistakable public demand to be involved in the process. Submissions in response to the first document stressed the need for broad consultation in order for the public to have the opportunity to influence further policy developments.[4] They also attached great importance to fully informing people about proposed changes, and to making decisions, and the justification for those decisions, public.[4]

Who has been involved? The annual reports state that there have been numerous consultations with individuals and groups of all types. These have included expert lay people, such as those used in the consensus approaches, as well as attendees at meetings and *hui*, and individuals and organisations submitting responses to discussion documents. There was, in the 1993 report, an awareness that the consultation process was not reaching all groups in the community,[11] and late in 1993 a series of ethics workshops were held involving older people, people with disabilities, those living in rural areas, urban dwellers on low incomes, Maori, Pacific Island people and teenagers.[12] In 1994 a further consultation initiative used randomly recruited members of the public.[12] It does appear, therefore, that the consultation process is attempting to hear as many different "voices" as it can.

The Committee appears to have consulted the public on a variety of issues. These have included the broad framework for priority setting, the results of consensus conferences, the broad set of priorities and the social values to be incorporated in priority setting. In fact, consultation appears to be carried out at almost every level of the priority-setting process. It is difficult to know, however, how much this consultation has influenced priorities where there has not already been an intention to make something a priority. It is also questionable whether public consultation has, at times, been dispensed with – for example, the reclassification of "integrated community care services" to "Maori health", which was merely stated to be a confirmation of the priorities set previously (see above).

Consultation has taken a variety of formats, each of which aim to listen to different voices. As well as public meetings, public forums, *hui* and consensus conferences, there has been the publication of three documents that aim both to broaden the debate and to acquire information about public views on priority setting: *The best of health. Deciding on the health services we value most*,[14] *Seeking Consensus*[13] and *The best of health 2: How we decide on the health and disability services we value most*.[15] Apart from these published documents, however, it is not clear how much, or what, information has been provided to those consulted about priorities.

In New Zealand the emphasis of the consultation process appears in all areas to be on acquiring many differing views and then attempting to obtain consensus rather than attempting to aggregate views and thus "flatten them out" (see Chapter 8). Consultation seems to have been a successful part of the priority-setting process to date. Despite this appearance of success the Committee has expressed concern that the public should not feel that it is being overconsulted. This is particularly so given that other authorities, for example the New Zealand Regional Health Authorities, are also consulting the public about health care provision. The core services report for 1994 stresses this point, especially where changes to services are not immediately apparent following consultation.[12] (See Chapter 8 for further discussion about commitment to change following consultation.)

From the literature produced by the Core Services Committee, consultation with the public appears to have been, in general, a success. Because precise methods have not been described in detail, however, it is difficult either to discern from the reports how methodological difficulties have been resolved, or on a more sceptical note, whether they have been ignored. If some of the many difficulties have been resolved, it would be useful for those elsewhere to be able to learn from the experience of New Zealand. If, however, the methodological problems have been ignored, it is difficult to know how much value can be attributed to the results obtained by this priority-setting exercise.

ELEMENTS OF TECHNICAL PRIORITY SETTING: THE DESIRE FOR A FRAMEWORK OF PRINCIPLES

Responses to the initial consultation document about core services[4,5] stated that the priority-setting process should begin with debate about the philosophical, ethical and moral basis that core services should have. Even with a system based on bargaining and consensus, it seems to have been clear to many that there should be a general framework of objectives within which priorities could be set. Ensuring fairness/universal access to basic services seems to have been the overriding principle for many,[4,6] and the subsequent framework developed by the Committee reflects this notion, at least in its titles. The four principles outlined in *The best of health 2* are "What are the benefits?", "Is it value for money?", "Is it fair?" and "Is it consistent with the community's values and priorities?"[15] What is meant by "Is it fair?" is not entirely clear. It is interesting that by far the most emphasis in *The best of health 2* is given to this question,[15] yet the section concentrates almost exclusively on, at a personal level, the question of relative benefit compared with cost! This is essentially an efficiency, rather than an equity, question – which would be implied by the title "is it fair?" In the subsequent report by the committee, however, the question of fairness is treated quite differently, being related to issues of regional equity and equity between socio-economic groups.[12]

It is interesting to compare the principles chosen by the New Zealand Core Services Committee with those developed by the Dutch Government Committee on Choices in Health Care.[3] In the Netherlands priority setting is seen as occurring through a "sieve" which will retain care which is unnecessary, ineffective, inefficient, or which can be left to individual responsibility (*Choices in Health Care*,[3] pp.84–87). These frameworks are therefore similar in content, with both containing effectiveness and cost-effectiveness as basic principles.

The effect that New Zealand's philosophical framework will have on the assessment of core services is not completely clear, although it is recommended that these principles should be taken into account in the purchasing decisions taken by RHAs.[12] In fact, the framework is very broad, and may well just provide a background to the work of the Committee within more specific objectives. The Committee undoubtedly feels that the framework provides them with a basis for their deliberations.[12] The framework may also provide a useful basis against which to measure the success of the Committee's work in priority setting.

CONCLUSION: THE IMPLICATIONS FROM NEW ZEALAND

In New Zealand priority setting has been based on consensus: essentially, a political process has been developed whereby clinical and lay views together inform the decisions that are made. This emphasis on the bargaining process pervades the whole of the approach by the Core Services Committee, with, at different levels, both different mixes of lay and clinical viewpoints and the inclusion of different "publics" in the decision process. Although essentially a bargaining approach, however, there are elements of technical methodologies apparent in the framework generated by the Core Services Committee.

How useful would this approach be elsewhere? Ham has suggested that the New Zealand approach to priority setting seems much more appropriate to the UK setting than that of Oregon.[18] It is certainly easier to imagine the application of rationing of the New Zealand kind in the UK health care system, than the technical rationing of Oregon. Organisational factors within health care systems will be a major element in determining the form of priority setting which is most appropriate for any society. The similarity of the national health care systems in New Zealand and the UK would imply that the Core Services process could work in the UK. Another important element is the social acceptability of rationing. A clear rejection of the Oregon approach in New Zealand is mirrored in the UK, with a similar aversion to technical rationing schemes evident in publications in both countries.[5,19]

It is of note, however, that New Zealand's approach to priority setting has been much less publicised worldwide than that of Oregon. The public, professional and academic reaction has been both much more limited and much less vehement. Further, the potential for using similar plans elsewhere has received relatively little discussion. The approach generated in New Zealand is far less radical than that of Oregon, with the nature of the exercise being one of gradual incremental change from the status quo. Although New Zealand's reports indicate that change is beginning to occur as a result of their attempts to set priorities explicitly, the danger inherent in such plans is that this change could be merely illusory. The endless consultation may just provide the facade for a continuation of the age-old story of implicit rationing by clinicians. While the attractiveness of this plan to other societies will probably lie in its flexibility, its very malleability may prove to be its downfall as a means of explicit priority setting.

REFERENCES

1. Klein R. Dimensions of rationing: who should do what? *BMJ* 1993; **307**: 309-11.
2. Seedhouse D. Core health services – a fiction? *N Z Med J* 1993; **106**: 8.
3. Government Committee on Choices in Health Care. *Choices in Health Care*. Ministry of Welfare, Health and Cultural Affairs, Rijswijk, 1992.
4. The Bridgeport Group. *The core debate. Stage one: how we define the core. Review of submissions*. Department of Health, Wellington, New Zealand, 1992.
5. Minister of Health (New Zealand). *The core debate. Stage one: how we define the core*. Minister of Health, Wellington, New Zealand, 1991.
6. National Advisory Committee on Core Health and Disability Support Services. *Core Health and Disability Support Services for 1993/94*. National Advisory Committe on Core Health and Disability Support Services, Wellington, New Zealand, 1992.
7. Anon. Public consultation – ethics workshops. *The Core Debater* 1994; **1**: 4.
8. Anon. Public forums – the public's opinion. *The Core Debater* 1994; **3**: 7.
9. Anon. Who should get treatment first – what the public thinks. *The Core Debater* 1995; **4**: 2–4.
10. National Advisory Committee on Core Health and Disability Support Services. *A report on the public forums held to discuss priority criteria setting for cataract removal and coronary artery bypass grafting*. National Advisory Committee on Core Health and Disability Support Services, Wellington, New Zealand, 1994.
11. National Advisory Committee on Core Health and Disability Support Services. *Core Services for 1994/95*. National Advisory Committee on Core Health and Disability Support Services, Wellington, New Zealand, 1993.
12. National Advisory Committee on Core Health and Disability Support Services. *Core Services for 1995/6*. National Advisory Committee on Core Health and Disability Support Services, Wellington, New Zealand, 1994.
13. National Advisory Committee on Core Health and Disability Support Services. *Seeking consensus*. National Advisory Committee on Core Health and Disability Support Services, Wellington, New Zealand, 1993.
14. National Advisory Committee on Core Health and Disability Support Services. *The best of health. Deciding on the health services we value most*. Department of Health, Wellington, New Zealand, 1992.
15. National Advisory Committee on Core Health and Disability Support

Services. *The best of health 2. How we decide on the health and disability support services we value most.* National Advisory Committee on Core Health and Disability Support Services, Wellington, New Zealand, 1994.

16. Jones L. Editorial. *The Core Debater* 1994; **1**: 1–2.
17. Anon. Core services committee rejects 'simple list' approach to define publicly funded services for New Zealanders. *The Core Debater* 1994; **3**: 1–2.
18. Ham C. Health care rationing. *BMJ* 1995; **310**: 1483–4.
19. Health Committee. *Priority setting in the NHS: purchasing. Volume 1.* HMSO, London, 1995.

CHAPTER FOUR

IAN HARVEY

Philosophical Perspectives on Priority Setting

It may not immediately be apparent why, when the subject under consideration is that of priority setting and when the ambition is to produce practical recommendations for action, there should be a chapter devoted to moral philosophy. The reason lies in the fact that, despite philosophy's reputation as an abstract pursuit (itself a parody), there are increasing numbers of philosophers whose primary interest is in applied issues, particularly in the fields of health, social and legal policy. Such philosophers undertake the practical tasks of dissecting out and critically examining the ideas that underpin often heated debates about which course of action is "ethical" in a particular situation. One area of health care in which this critical examination can be undertaken is that of priority setting.

The philosophical approach outlined in this chapter aims for greater clarity by making *explicit* those assumptions and beliefs which are often merely *implicit* in discussion. One underlying purpose is that individuals with conflicting views may, without necessarily resolving those differences, none the less develop – through the process of critically analysing ideas – a more sensitive appreciation of existing diversity. Further, the chapter provides the real context for the debate about priority setting, and the views held by the different participants in this debate.

Priority Setting: The Health Care Debate.
Edited by J. Coast, J. Donovan and S. Frankel.   © 1996 John Wiley & Sons Ltd.

The chapter begins by describing the tensions between the different ethical bases from which the priority-setting debate can be conducted. Two main ethical models which offer guidance to those interested in priority setting are discussed. The first emphasises the interpersonal aspects of the relationship between health workers and patients, and attaches special importance to respect for the autonomy of patients: it is known as the deontological model. The second model, consequentialism – and in particular its subcategory utilitarianism – emphasises the importance of maximising the happiness or utility that accrues from health care. A third vital element – a concern for equity – is also discussed. The potential conflicts that may arise between the strict utilitarian goal of utility maximisation and the goal of equity are also considered.

The chapter then analyses the conflicting beliefs and behaviour of health care workers on the one hand and of health economists on the other against the background of their ethical principles. This analysis suggests that all groups derive their ethical approaches from a varying mixture of the available ethical models. Although severe practical difficulties persist – not the least of these being the outright rejection by a number of health professionals of the necessity for priority setting/rationing within the NHS – the chapter raises hope that the polarised and stereotypical views often expressed in the debate about priority setting may be more rhetorical than truly reflective of underlying beliefs. It thus raises the potential for accepting that conflict exists, but moving beyond this conflict to find a way forward for priority setting.

ETHICS IN HEALTH CARE

Medical ethics has been defined by Gillon as "an analytic activity in which the concepts, assumptions, beliefs, attitudes, emotions, reasons, and arguments underlying medicomoral decision making are examined critically".[1] He also suggests certain activities that fall outside this definition – in particular the drawing up and enforcing of professional codes of conduct (although such "ethical" codes should be rooted in some guiding moral principle(s)). Equally he excludes from his definition those "sociological/psychological/ anthropological/historical efforts to discover the attitudes, mores or ethos of a particular community".[1] In other words Gillon properly focuses upon moral philosophy, and its subsidiary subject medical ethics, as the critical analysis of *ideas*, removed from their social context. Medical ethics is not *itself* a social science.

Whilst this may be true, ethical concepts are plainly adopted and used differently by different groups in society and it is essential to attempt to describe some of these social patterns, alongside the purely philosophical issues. To omit this would render it virtually impossible to make practical recommendations. Some of what follows is therefore concerned less with pure moral philosophy than with what has been loosely called "ethnoethics",[2,3] which involves the comparative study and appreciation of moral systems both between and within societies. A joint consideration of both ethical models and their social context may well, in the long run, prove more productive in the practical matter of developing widely acceptable health policies in the UK, than an excessive concentration upon moral theories in isolation.

Many of those more formally engaged in the debate about the shape of the health service, about public preferences and about the allocation of scarce resources – a mixture of academics, practitioners and managers – extol the virtues of being more *explicit* about decision-making, of opening to public scrutiny the informal rules that operate unacknowledged. To this extent their desires and those of medical ethicists coincide. Both groups are concerned to lay bare the process of reasoning that underpins actions. Moral reasoning has indeed been said to consist of four stages:[4]

- Clarification – defining exactly what the moral problem is.
- Drawing upon moral theories in order to identify the moral principles and rules that pertain to the situation.
- Stating arguments favouring or opposing the various rules so derived.
- Providing clear guidance for practice and behaviour.

Moral reasoning, expressed in these terms, is a type of structured approach to problem analysis that will be recognisable to many non-philosophers. It is arguably a basic analytical tool in any debate about the shape of health services, and educational initiatives may well be needed to remedy a general lack of skill and appreciation in this area. But a critical limitation of the method must also be recognised, that is, that "moral reasoning provides no rational way, no indisputable algorithm, by which to choose between conflicting moral theories or principles".[4] While it can certainly illuminate the issues,[5] moral reasoning provides no incontestable way of choosing between conflicting ethical models. The favouring of one ethical system above another thus remains a wholly subjective, value-laden judgement. There is no logical way of resolving differences of ethical perspective except in so far as structured debate may lead to identification of inconsistencies, appreciation of others' viewpoints, and perhaps ultimately to convergence of thinking.

ETHICAL MODELS – HELP OR HINDRANCE?

It is possible to "do" moral philosophy – the critical analysis of ideas about human conduct – without seeking to develop overarching models or theories of how we ought to conduct ourselves. It is possible to argue that we should approach each problem separately and keep theorising to a minimum. There is indeed a strongly held view in philosophical circles that the development of all-embracing theories represents a fatally flawed attempt to emulate the natural sciences. This approach has been referred to disparagingly as an "engineering model" of applied ethics[6] in which theories have the undesirable effect of exerting strong normative pressures and thus tend to constrain thought along one of a restricted number of pathways.[7,8]

However justified such criticism may be, and however much a concentration upon these models may insidiously contribute to a counterproductive polarisation in the debate about priorities in health care, it is important to review them. Partly this is because they are already well known – at least in outline – and partly because, however stereotypic they may be, they represent a genuine strand in the daily thinking of many engaged in health care provision and in health care policy making. Thus, they impinge upon the approaches to priority setting favoured by these different individuals.

DEONTOLOGY AND CONSEQUENTIALISM

The two principal ethical models to be considered are *deontology* and *consequentialism*. These are examples of *technical ethics* (carefully considered ethical principles whose implications have been subjected to rigorous scrutiny), which may be distinguished from *everyday ethics* – our intuitive and spontaneous ethical reactions to daily situations. Plainly, however, there is likely to be substantial overlap between the technical and the everyday. Furthermore, both models represent examples of *persisting ethics* (overarching theories which can in principle be applied to all situations) – to be distinguished from *specific/dramatic ethics*, whose application is confined to particular discrete situations, such as whether to cease feeding patients in vegetative states.[9,10] Once again there is substantial overlap between the persisting and the specific.

DEONTOLOGY

Deriving from the Greek word *deon* (duty), this ethical model asserts that in judging an action we should be principally concerned *not* with the actual *consequences* (or *outcome*) of the action but with whether the person acted according to a perceived duty and *intended* some good to occur. Under this model there are certain duties which should be performed *regardless of the consequences*.[9] Historically Immanuel Kant (1724–1804) is probably the best known exponent of a deontological approach. Kant's supreme moral law proposes, amongst other things, that no person should be treated only as a means but always as an end. In other words, and this is a critical point in understanding the deontological approach, it is wrong totally to ignore one's duties to one individual for the sake of the greater good of other individuals. Menzel[11] has strikingly illustrated Kant's central point using a dilemma from fiction (Dostoyevsky, *The Brothers Karamazov*), to which a true deontologist's unequivocating response would be in the negative:

> Imagine that to make all men eternally happy it was essential to torture to death only one tiny creature – a baby beating its breast with its fist – . . . and to found that edifice on its unavenged tears. Would you consent to be the architect . .?

Kant provides a further criterion (the *categorical imperative*) by which "right" action should be judged, namely that one should "act only on the maxim which you can at the same time will to be universal law". Crudely paraphrased, this means that you should do to others what you would have them do to you.

CONSEQUENTIALISM

This group of moral theories holds that it is only by the *consequences* of actions that they can be judged to be right or wrong. The relevant consequence that is taken into consideration may be one of any number of possible outcomes and varies between subcategories of consequentialism.

Utilitarianism, amongst whose principal exponents in the nineteenth century were Jeremy Bentham and John Stuart Mill, is a variant of consequentialism with the following characteristics. First it considers happiness (often substituted – although it is not self-evident that the concepts are interchangeable – by the terms "utility" or "welfare" by many who consider themselves, and are considered by others to be, utilitarians) to be the relevant outcome. Second, the morally right action is to seek to maximise the quantity of that outcome experienced by mankind – "the greatest happiness of the greatest number", in Bentham's famous but ambiguous aphorism.[12] A more sophisticated contemporary formulation of utilitarianism is that it involves maximising the "satisfaction of individuals' autonomous preferences".[1] This inclines more towards utility than happiness as the relevant consequence of interest. It should be emphasised, however, that there are non-utilitarian consequentialists who differ from utilitarians either in not focusing upon *utility* as the outcome of interest or in not seeking to *maximise* the quantity of their chosen outcome or who differ in both respects.

Other outcomes apart from happiness and utility have indeed been proposed as relevant in framing health care policy. These include social value (a judgement regarding the usefulness of individuals to society), accumulated earnings, projected additional length of life, and number of lives saved. These all differ more or less subtly from maximisation of utility.[13] Although ethicists have been inclined to dismiss these alternative consequences, they are not simply theoretical alternatives. They have achieved a certain currency in particular health care rationing decisions. Accumulated earnings have, at times, contributed to benefit estimation in the widely used economic technique of cost–benefit analysis. Social value was a consequence explicitly considered by the Admissions and Policy Committee of the Swedish hospital in Seattle, USA in the early days of renal dialysis. Consisting of lay members and clinicians, this committee established and applied criteria for inclusion in the (then) scarce dialysis programme. These criteria included an estimate of the social worth (based on involvement in such things as church and community activities) of candidates for dialysis.[14] Others have suggested that in many situations the number of lives saved is likely to be the outcome of overwhelming interest, a view graphically labelled in the United States the "Rule of Rescue".[15]

LOCATING THE HEALTH POLICY DEBATE

Clearly there are profound differences between the deontological and consequentialist (particularly the utilitarian) ethical models. Not only does this difference constitute a dividing line in moral, social and political philosophy[16] but its effects reverberate in the parallel practical worlds of social and health policy. Many of the conflicting views expressed in public and political debate about health and social policy have their (usually unacknowledged) roots in these differing ethical approaches. Many individuals draw inspiration from both ethical models, and most of us – to at least some degree – alternate between them according to circumstance. Although the divide may, on closer scrutiny, prove to be an example of what Douglas Black has called a "false antithesis",[17] the passions frequently generated are none the less real. Arguably, amongst the greatest practical challenges facing those interested in health policy and priority setting is the need to encourage health practitioners, policy makers and the electorate at large to analyse and reflect upon the ethical, social and historical origins of their beliefs and practices.

Some observers of health services have proposed that it is legitimate to generalise about the ethical approaches of different social groups.

Doctors on the one hand and economists on the other have come under particularly close scrutiny and it is a view commonly held that their ethical approaches represent the opposite ends of a moral spectrum. Rutten, for example, has suggested, without endorsing the view, that a common perception is that:

> . . . medical ethics is very much concerned with the individualistic considerations of virtue and duty and that it tends to emphasise the need for the individual doctor to do his utmost for the individual patient. The objective of economics is utilitarian and economists strive to maximise benefits to society given the resources available.[18]

This assessment of the differences between doctors' and economists' perceptions encapsulates the distinction already discussed between deontology and utilitarianism. But is this a valid assessment? Is the difference as stark as this? If there is any truth in the description, are there relevant contextual factors which may enhance our understanding and provide some possibility of convergence? And spreading the focus further afield, are these differing views, if they exist, confined only to medicine and economics? To answer these points one needs to examine in more detail the viewpoints of health professionals on the one hand and of economists on the other against the backdrop of the fundamental ethical models already described.

DEONTOLOGY AND THE PRACTICE OF HEALTH CARE

Even a cursory examination of the many codes of conduct that have been formulated over the years to regulate medical practice reveals strong deontological elements.[19] Most contain some rules about the manner in which doctors should treat their patients (as ends, not means) which make no reference to consequences. Several reasons may be proposed as to why this should be so.

First, an elaboration of rules of conduct based on deontology has accompanied the professionalisation and rising status of many health care groups – medicine, nursing and midwifery – during the nineteenth and early twentieth centuries. In the case of medicine in Britain these rules developed under the auspices of a statutory body

– the General Medical Council, established in 1858.[20,21] It seems clear that one device that has been widely employed over many years, seemingly to enhance the social standing of an occupation, is the adoption of a more or less elaborate code of conduct that emphasises, in general terms, duties and standards of integrity, confidentiality and honesty. Many other occupations within the health care sector have followed doctors and repeated this process of adopting ethical codes with strong deontological overtones. This raises the interesting question of why this pattern should have been repeated. Is it perhaps the case that a wide range of professional groups have arrived, by different routes, at a common perception – namely, that society at large attaches a premium to a display of deontological concern and commitment? Does society at large expect that groups it deems "professions" will display towards their clients forms of concern which are more complex and multifaceted than the desire simply to produce measurable benefit?

A number of discrete historical events have also been crucial in the rise of deontology in medicine. In particular the involvement of doctors in eugenic and other experiments in Nazi Germany and the United States,[22] and their complicity in the incarceration in psychiatric hospitals of political prisoners in the Soviet Union, created widespread revulsion during this century against medical involvement in governmental manipulation of the population. Deontology seemed, with its emphasis upon treating individuals as "ends", to provide a powerful buttress against a recurrence of such state-sponsored atrocities.[23] Several ethical codes dominated by deontological exhortations were developed and promulgated in the years after 1945 as a direct result of reaction against this earlier behaviour.[1]

A third reason identified as encouraging deontology amongst health professionals stems from the patient's allegedly poor understanding of the health care which they need to "consume" in order to achieve better health. The patient, it is argued, is bound to lack the technical knowledge required to make sound judgements and thus is forced to hand over property rights in his or her health to the doctor.[24] A deontological ethical code, it is argued, reassures the patient that the health professional will act as an agent in *that patient's* best interests.

CONSEQUENTIALISM AND THE PRACTICE OF HEALTH CARE

Turning to the other side of the discussion, to what extent can consequentialist elements be discerned in medical thinking and practice? Most ethical codes certainly contain both the deontological and the consequentialist. The Hippocratic Oath, for example, requires the doctor to "follow that system or regimen which, according to my ability and judgement I consider for the benefit of my patients". Plainly the word "benefit" carries strong consequentialist overtones. The doctor's actions, it suggests, are to be judged by results as well as by the personal integrity with which he/she acts. The widely commended principles of *beneficence* and *non-maleficence* (doing good and not doing harm) are also intrinsically consequentialist and feature prominently as criteria by which ethical medical practice is judged. No more stark statement of a consequentialist – but certainly not a utilitarian – view could be found than Levinsky's:

> . . . Physicians are required *to do everything that they believe may benefit each patient* [my italics] without regard to costs or other societal considerations.[25]

THE INDIVIDUAL VERSUS THE SOCIETAL

Levinsky's statement leads towards other relevant issues in considering the moral positions of economists and health workers. It is clear from what has been said that health workers function within an ethical framework that has both *deontological* and *consequentialist* characteristics. But statements such as Levinsky's, which a significant number of practitioners would probably support,[26] suggest that they are prepared only to consider the consequences for their own patients. In other words their consequentialist focus is narrow and their orientation overwhelmingly individualistic. Utilitarians aim, by contrast and by definition, to maximise utility across society. Their ethical base is societal[4]. How valid a characterisation is this?

There are in fact many discrete instances where doctors have participated in choosing between patients in such a way that the patient in front of them did not automatically take priority. In so doing wider criteria and concerns are brought into play.[27] The simplest example involves the actions of clinicians in wartime, where the practice of triage selects those patients for whom immediate intervention can produce most benefit.[14] Other potential patients are left either because their problems are irremediable or because they will not suffer from delay. Similar principles of triage have been introduced, with overt medical involvement, in civil disaster planning and to the routine work practices of many hospital Accident and Emergency departments. Even the categorisation of outpatient referrals into urgent and non-urgent cases is an aspect of the weighing in the balance of competing interests and needs of patients. Surgeons are well aware that some of those judged non-urgent will spend prolonged periods waiting for treatment, during which time their suffering will continue and in some instances they may die. Gillon offers numerous further instances from primary care of doctors acknowledging that potentially beneficial interventions cannot always be offered to their own patients, either because of scarcity, cost or both.[28]

Expensive and scarce life-saving interventions have produced the clearest examples of health workers' willingness to choose between patients. Starting with penicillin during the 1940s, when its use was targeted upon soldiers rather than civilians, more recent examples exist – such as renal dialysis and organ transplantation – where doctors are closely involved in making uncomfortable choices between the presenting patient and other potential patients.[29] The limited availability of liver transplantation has led, for example, to prolonged discussion as to whether patients suffering from alcoholic liver disease should be recipients. Doctors have often chosen against such patients on the grounds that continued drinking may in time, amongst other things, damage the graft.[30] Better consequences for other non-alcoholic patients have led to a denial of potentially life-prolonging treatment for alcoholics. Similar arguments have occurred about coronary artery bypass grafting for smokers with coronary artery disease. These particular examples are potentially more complex than they might initially appear, however. The consequentialist argument has usually been couched in terms of only relative survival providing the basis upon which the liver transplantation choice has been made. But, as in the example of rationing of renal dialysis, there is a suspicion that medically held notions of social value and moral worth are significant features in these choices.[5] The general point is worth re-emphasising – that the outcome measure under consideration in consequentialist approaches is rarely simple and unidimensional.

The generalisation that doctors' moral choices always reflect a preference for the presenting patient over the concerns of a wider population of patients, known and unknown, is impossible to sustain.[31] Particular groups of doctors have shown themselves, in different societies and at different times, to be concerned about such issues as the aggregate life prolongation to be obtained from an intervention (liver transplantation), the aggregate social value of patients to society (early days of renal dialysis), and the opportunities foregone if practices are adopted which have only a small chance of producing benefit (taking throat swabs in all cases of sore throat, for example). The wider interests of the whole population of potential beneficiaries have in these instances been elevated above the interests of single patients. But even this statement has to be qualified. In the field of renal transplantation, for example, the imbalance that exists in the movement of cadaver kidneys between regions of the UK ("imports and exports") has led to great concern amongst transplant surgeons. Some regions have been perceived as importing an excessive number from other regions. One interpretation of this disquiet is that it reflects a sense of loyalty on the part of transplant surgeons to potential recipients in their own region that appears to surpass their concern for the wider population of potential recipients throughout the UK.

CONSEQUENTIALISM IN HEALTH POLICY AND HEALTH ECONOMICS

It is widely felt that health and social policy makers, given their aggregate concerns, are inclined to view potential solutions to problems in terms of aggregate effects (or consequences) and are less likely to be swayed by deontological concerns. But is there a uniform consequentialist view current amongst those formulating health policy? The answer must be in the negative. There are several strands within that tradition. One strand considers that social policy should be drawn up in such a way as to achieve an *optimal level of utility* from public expenditure. This has been called *preference* or *welfare utilitarianism*.[16] But other strands, exemplified historically by the Beveridge Report of 1942, aim for less than optimum utility and temper concern for utility enhancement with a concern, at least as strong, for the *distribution of benefits* within society. Beveridge's famous focus of attack was on the five giants of Want, Disease, Ignorance, Squalor and Idleness, and a cornerstone of his remedy was the principle of universal insurance coverage. He was attacked for this by welfare economists, in terms that have been repeated more recently, for his failure to *target* resources so as to achieve the maximum possible improvement in his chosen parameters.[32] Within this broad zone there are therefore varying perceptions of the objective being sought.

How do contemporary health economists fit into this taxonomy? More specifically, to what extent do they advocate utility *optimisation*? The record provides a varied picture, with different emphases placed upon the relative importance of utility optimisation (efficiency) on the one hand and upon concerns about distribution (equity) on the other. Mooney and Drummond, for example, suggest that "economics is about getting *better* value from the deployment of scarce resources" [emphasis added].[33] Mooney and Jensen[34] acknowledge the distributive consideration when they write:

> Classical utilitarianism may . . . fail if it does not attempt to take account of distributional issues. If cost–benefit analyses ignore these they may fail to reflect the importance that citizens get from knowing that their health service is concerned with distributional issues. That is not a circular argument. Any other simply omits an important source of value in modern health care systems.[34]

Mooney has also commented that :

> Allocative efficiency is not the sole criterion that health services are likely to adopt in deciding how to prioritise.[35]

Elsewhere, however, Mooney and McGuire[24] present a slightly different emphasis by stating that "the end sought by economic policy – *the maximisation of benefits* – is based upon an aggregation of . . . the utility derived . . . from the resource allocation process" [emphasis added]. Culyer has suggested that : ". . . the objective of health services is to promote health and, moreover, to do so in such a fashion as to maximise the impact on the nation's health of whatever resources are available to this end".[36] Alan Maynard's statement of purpose is arguably the closest to strict welfare utilitarianism. Having defined inefficiency as a situation in which costs are not minimised and benefits are not maximised, he proposes quite simply that "Inefficiency is unethical".[37] From a brief review of health economists' own statements of purpose it is clear that there is significant heterogeneity, ranging from utility optimisation to less strict forms of consequentialism which attach importance to equity considerations.

The discussion up to this point has placed two major groups – doctors and health economists – interested in the shape of health services, in the context of the two principal relevant ethical systems. There are certain other issues, not inherently ethical, that none the less impinge upon the continuing health policy debate. The first of these has to do with whether it is necessary to make choices at all between various possible interventions and programmes. At the heart of this is the question of whether resources are in fact scarce, since, if they are not, all interventions can be afforded and choices are thus unnecessary.

Resources – Scarce or Not?

It is axiomatic within economics that resources are scarce and hence choices are inevitable. Economics concerns itself centrally with describing and recommending approaches to the allocation of scarce resources. One could argue that it is not in fact essential to accept this axiom in order to be considered a utilitarian, since a utilitarian is simply one who judges the rightness or wrongness of an act by the extent to which it produces "happiness". It is not implicit in this that the means to produce happiness are scarce. But leaving these theoretical considerations to one side, how do different groups respond to the notion of scarce resources?

Moral philosophers have certainly become interested in examining the varied responses to this axiom amongst those working in health care. Winslow has pointed out that whilst scarcity on the battlefield and the need for choices in the form of triage have never seriously been challenged by doctors, it is constantly challenged in civilian medicine.[14] What is the morally relevant difference? Could it be, he suggests, that scarcity on the battlefield is seen as resulting from some natural disaster beyond any reasonable control, whereas civilian scarcity is seen as due to human failing or design? Or, put another way, the battlefield is seen, perhaps, as the setting for a "zero-sum" game where the available resources are fixed and gainers must be balanced by losers. Other settings, by contrast, are not seen as inherently "zero-sum" and the size of the cake is not perceived to be fixed.[14] If this generalisation is accepted, two possible logical explanations exist. The first is that doctors believe that the resources available to society are in principle infinite. Philosophers have commented that occasionally a total denial of scarcity is encountered – amongst both professionals and lay people – resulting in the view that there is no need to develop priorities, since all can be treated and there are no opportunities foregone even by expenditure that confers no benefit.[13] All that should be avoided under this "plentiful approach" is expenditure that does harm. This "plentiful" view will to many, however, seem absurd.

The second explanation is that doctors believe that the *proportion* of wealth that is given over to health care, particularly in relatively low spending countries such as the UK, is inadequate. If this is the perception, as seems inherently more likely, it is not the axiom of scarcity that is rejected but the size of the allocation given over to health, which is viewed as being the result of deliberate (usually governmental) policy. We should, so this argument runs, defer consideration of choices within health care until higher level choices have been made as between patterns of public and private expenditure, and between different forms of public expenditure. This point, even when made by doctors, is often couched in broadly utilitarian terms, contrasting the allegedly better value for money resulting from health spending with that accruing from other, supposedly less "efficient", forms of public expenditure.[38] A variant of this view is that the moment when choices and rationing may be necessary can be further deferred simply by ceasing to provide all ineffective medical and nursing interventions. Advocates of this approach argue that the resources thus released would be so sizeable that choices between the remaining, effective interventions would be unnecessary. This is an approach that has considerable appeal to governments for whom use of the term "rationing" carries political risks.[39] Others might feel that the act of denying ineffective interventions is in itself an act of priority setting and hence of rationing.

Differences of perception about resource scarcity need much closer examination, since it is upon such fundamental disagreements – which are sometimes merely misunderstandings resulting from a failure to use language precisely – that the whole further discussion about the need for rationing and priority setting, and about the voices that should be heard in that process, can founder. Recent evidence of marked polarisation on this point is provided by the outcome of a debate that preceded a national conference entitled "Priority Setting in the Health Service". Doctors and other health professionals split evenly (68 for, 65 against) on a motion: "This house believes that healthcare rationing is inevitable".[40] Almost half the health professionals present clearly rejected the current or future necessity for choices to be made in health care provision, in stark contrast to the views likely to be held by health economists and health service managers. In such circumstances it is extraordinarily difficult to develop further any discussion about priority setting.

The Tools of Health Economics

While the specific techniques and measurement instruments of health economics will not be considered in detail in this section, there are certain relevant issues that must be discussed. This is particularly so because some moral philosophers have become interested in examining in closer detail the way in which some of these measures relate to the wider ethical systems that have already been discussed. In particular, and surprisingly at first sight, measures of the Quality-Adjusted Life-Year (QALY) type (see Chapter 6) have been a source of dispute between their advocates on the one hand and, on the other, certain moral philosophers who in fact consider themselves to be utilitarians. How has this come about?

These utilitarian philosophers have been critical of QALY-type measures in two key respects. The first point of criticism has been that they are based upon indirectly obtained utility values – values not from subjects actually experiencing the impaired state of health under consideration but instead from more or less representative samples from various populations. This, it is argued, violates the principle that utilitarianism seeks to maximise the *autonomous preferences of individuals* (see above) and substitutes rather the vicarious preferences of unaffected individuals. The justifications for this approach have been of two types. First, on the grounds of practicality, it has been argued that it is neither feasible nor necessary to canvass the views of each and every category of patient, especially as the QALY is intended to provide only general policy guidance. The second argument has been that those who, by paying taxes, fund public health services are entitled to influence the pattern of expenditure that they may expect to receive in the future, even if they are well at present. This argument implicitly contains a libertarian view of taxation – specifically that in return for shouldering the burden of taxation the taxpayer should be able to exercise significant control over the uses to which those resources are put.[41] The contrary argument has been that, putting to one side considerations about the need to respect each patient's autonomy, within a utilitarian framework it is the valuation put upon life and its quality by the affected individual that matters and not that of a third party.[42]

The second objection has centred upon the fact that under QALY-type approaches utility is multiplied by time to give a utility-years measure of benefit. This is held to violate the Benthamite principle that everybody counts for one and nobody for more than one. The young, it is argued, have an intrinsically greater chance of accumulating QALYs than the elderly, simply because young people with a given condition will on average live longer than someone older with the same condition. Were QALYs to be used in allocating resources the young would thereby be favoured over the elderly. The charge that is being levelled is essentially that of "ageism".[43]

DEONTOLOGY AND CONSEQUENTIALISM: IS A UNIFYING MODEL POSSIBLE?

Whilst health workers are without doubt concerned about the consequences of their actions (in terms of doing good, or being beneficent), and many are demonstrably willing to take account of the effect of their actions on a constituency wider than simply their own patients, they are in general unsympathetic towards strict welfare utilitarianism. It seems for one thing to carry the risk that deontological concerns about integrity will always be subservient to the utility-optimising requirement of strict utilitarianism. Is it possible to accommodate this concern within a single overarching ethical model? Various arguments have been proposed to try to achieve this. One version has been to defend the special relationship and special obligations between doctor and patient by asserting that these distinct interpersonal attributes themselves produce utility – so called *process* utility[24] – and that without them, utility will remain suboptimal.[28,44] Expressed slightly differently, it is suggested that total (aggregate) utility is the sum of utility which arises from the consequences of actions (outcome utility) and utility which flows from the manner in which those consequences are achieved (process utility). What this formulation achieves – and needless to say it is not universally accepted – is to represent deontological concerns as a special type of utility within a utilitarian framework. In practice, whilst this is theoretically attractive, it fails to satisfy a more fundamental objection to utilitarianism articulated by some deontologists – namely their rejection of the whole utilitarian calculus, and of the empirical possibility of determining the moral rightness of actions in such a way.[45]

THE THIRD VITAL ELEMENT – EQUITY

Incorporating particular deontological concerns about integrity and honesty into a unified utility-optimising schema (see above) ignores a third attribute of moral behaviour which has been mentioned but not yet fully considered – distributive concerns, also known as *equity* or *justice*. A fundamental aspect of deontology is expressed in Kant's Categorical Imperative – act only in a way that you could envisage being applied universally, including to yourself – which expresses a notion of consistency or evenness of behaviour. Many deontological critics of utilitarianism have expressed anxiety at its potential impact upon the distribution of health care, and in particular at the lack of explicit interest in issues of equity.[11,14,34] The basic dilemma may be expressed as follows. Should one seek to optimise utility *without regard* to the pattern of distribution of that utility across identifiable groups within society – such as age groups, the sexes, social classes, and so on?

Several medical ethicists have analysed this problem. Winslow, for example, argues for the limitation of utilitarian considerations and for the establishment of a basic presumption in favour of equity, by which he means equal access to health care for those in equal need.[14] He commends the Harvard philosopher John Rawls' theory of justice as a coherent model of a just society which achieves a defensible balance between utility and equality.[46] Rawls' theory has been much quoted in this connection and warrants closer consideration.

Rawls seeks to root his model of society firmly by asking us to imagine a group of rational decision-makers gathered together to create a society from scratch. They are all self-interested and equal. Moreover they operate behind a "veil of ignorance", by not knowing in advance how any of their decisions will affect them personally. He postulates, however, that these decision-makers will have knowledge of certain primary goods that any rational person would be expected to desire, including rights and liberties, opportunities and powers, income and wealth, and self-respect. Interestingly, good health and access to health care do not comprise one of these basic primary desires in Rawls' system, although this has not deterred health care philosophers from adopting his approach. Rawls argues that these rational participants would accept two fundamental principles, first that of equality in the assignment of basic rights and duties and second that social and economic inequalities would be accepted as just *only if they resulted in compensating benefits for everyone*. The second of these is known as the Maximin rule which states that "inequalities are permissible when they maximise . . . the long-term expectations of the least fortunate group in society".[46] Rawls further argues that the participants in this whole process would be most unlikely (because of the veil of ignorance) to propose a social organisation (as in principle a strict utilitarian might) in which a majority achieved great happiness, at the expense of an enslaved minority.

Rawls' theory thus leads us through a series of steps of intuitive reasoning to build a social structure on a base of various specified assumptions. Some have criticised Rawls' work as an attempt to construct a model using idealised assumptions about an unrealistically simple system.[47] Other philosophers of health care have drawn on it as the inspiration behind much of their thinking.

Yet some philosophers find the inequity implicit in Rawls' Maximin rule unacceptable.[48] Perhaps the most radical approach to the equity problem has been to suggest that chances for particular health care interventions should be distributed exactly equally by lottery.[13,43,49] This proposal has been supported particularly by those critical of QALYs. Having rejected, on the grounds of "ageism", the use of QALYs to choose between, for example, an 80-year-old and a 40-year-old requiring cardiac surgery, they propose that the toss of a coin provides the most equitable solution. On the whole, however, this solution – although intended as a serious contribution to the philosophical debate – has tended to be dismissed as merely a curiosity, particularly by health workers.

A strict utilitarian might respond to all that has been said about justice and equity by arguing as follows: all that is required in order to incorporate concerns about equity into the utilitarian model is to attach substantial negative utility to the iniquitous distribution of health care.[24] This parallels the approach adopted with regard to deontological concerns (see above). The overarching unified utilitarian system would thereby be restored. There are dangers, perhaps, in the endless elaboration of utilitarianism to incorporate deontological and distributive considerations. The first is the practical danger that the model will run far ahead of our actual abilities to develop and utilise appropriate measuring instruments. The tools in current use (such as the QALY) seek only to incorporate utilities relating to health status. We may be falsely reassured by knowing that we could *in principle*, and with sufficient time and effort, incorporate these elements of process utility, whilst continuing *in practice* to make decisions without them.

The second problem relates to the results that might emerge even if it were possible to ascertain the utility attached by the public to equity. What happens if the population does not value equitable distribution particularly highly? Those philosophers who attach great importance to it are unlikely to find this acceptable, since they prize equity as a morally correct attribute regardless of its popularity. If this were to be the case the apparent synthesis of utilitarian and distributive concerns would prove illusory. Some evidence already exists that the general population is inclined to weight differently the utilities of different social groups.[50] Utilitarians who support efforts to mirror the public's utilities as precisely as possible are likely to find themselves in continuing conflict with others for whom equity and justice are major, if not overriding, considerations.

In summary, therefore, three ethical concerns – expressed in deontology, consequentialism and justice – stand out as the peaks in the ethical terrain of relevance to priority setting in health services. It is mistaken too firmly to identify particular professional groups with particular ethical approaches, since significant heterogeneity exists within each. Indeed it is likely that each interested individual – to whichever broad grouping they belong – derives their ethical perspective from a changing combination of these three basic models. Few of us can aspire to behave in a manner consistent with only one ethical approach. Rather we may be thought of as moral chameleons, subtly, and often unconsciously, changing our positions and views in response to fluctuating moral surroundings.

CONSULTING THE PUBLIC ABOUT HEALTH CARE: THE MORAL ARGUMENTS

Many of the groups working in the NHS lay claim to being particularly sensitive and responsive to public wishes and derive some of their authority from those claims.[51] Such assertions do not, however, reveal the underlying moral arguments at work.

Deontologists argue that flowing logically from the Kantian requirement always to treat people as ends and not only as means and to act only in a way that can be made universal, comes a respect for the autonomy and wishes of individuals. Practically, this finds expression in a commitment to allow patients as much freedom as possible in making decisions about which medical and other interventions they receive. Two further points emerge from this. The first is that deontology, from the point of view of health professionals, is potentially a double-edged weapon. On the one hand it provides the basis from which the special characteristics of the doctor–patient relationship can be defended, but on the other it emphasises patient autonomy and rejects, except in exceptional circumstances, the paternalistic tendency of professionals to overrule or ignore patients' preferences.[5] The second point is that an emphasis upon autonomy attaches intrinsically greater importance to the views of actual patients than to those of individuals in good health who are merely potential future patients.[5] In this respect deontological reasoning leads to a similar conclusion to that of those utilitarians who object to QALY methodologies (see above) – namely that it is the views of actual sufferers which should be paramount.

In the case of utilitarianism there is a similar strong emphasis upon public participation in health care, founded in this instance upon the principle of maximising the additional utility which results from changes in health status. Professional paternalism is tolerated within this framework only in so far as it may be inevitable to some degree when individual patients cannot comprehend the implications of the alternatives before them. However, within the utilitarian perspective there is, as already discussed, divergence about the degree to which the general (tax-paying) public's utility values should be used as well as or instead of those of actual patients.

That there are strong moral arguments why health services and health professionals should submit in general to the preferences of the public is beyond doubt. How the "public" should be defined in this context (as between those who are ill and those who are well) is contested, however. Whether this commitment to public preferences is reached via a mainly deontological or mainly utilitarian route may be of importance in particular circumstances. Take as an example an intervention that is given high priority for funding by the public (both patients and others) but for which there is no evidence that it produces any measurable improvement in health status across a wide and comprehensive range of outcome measures. A strict utilitarian response to this situation might well argue that in the absence of evidence of measurable improvement in health and hence in health-related utility such an intervention should not be funded. A deontologist might well be inclined to argue differently, however, that not everything has value only as it contributes to maximising happiness or utility,[52] and that utilitarianism can successfully optimise the satisfaction of only a partial and incomplete set of human requirements for health care.[53] The satisfaction of the autonomously expressed wishes of the public, despite the lack of independent evidence of effectiveness, might be held, by a deontologist, to be sufficient reason to fund such an intervention.

NEEDS: THE MORAL ARGUMENTS

The needs-based model of priority setting itself has many facets (see Chapter 5). One of its commonest manifestations, however, is in the guise of the largely descriptive annual reports that are produced by Directors of Public Health within health authorities and health commissions in the UK. Such reports frequently contain large amounts of routine (and some ad hoc) data describing the patterns of mortality and morbidity within a defined population. These are put forward, with more or less conviction, as an attempt to shed some light upon the underlying needs of that population. How might a moral philosopher view such a claim?

A deontological response would be likely to focus upon the extent to which the needs identified were shaped by the availability of data and by the interpretation placed upon those data by authors with a specific professional background. Such an analysis would probably conclude that the approach in many cases is excessively rooted in a paternalistic definition of need, which places insufficient emphasis upon considerations of autonomy. The fact that limitations in the data available are as likely to be responsible is unlikely to weaken the objection. In this connection it must be acknowledged that some annual reports have gone to strenuous lengths to involve the wider public to the maximum possible degree in defining their scope and focus.

A strict utilitarian, by contrast, would be critical of this approach to priority setting for quite different reasons – namely, that if one's chosen objective is to maximise utility within available resources the traditional descriptive needs document is generally unhelpful. This is because such documents usually contain no consideration of the available interventions to tackle the needs described nor an assessment of their relative effectiveness and cost. Again it must be acknowledged that some annual reports have deliberately attempted to move in this direction.

RECOGNISING GRAINS OF TRUTH: PRACTICAL PROPOSALS FOR A MEETING OF MINDS

The picture that emerges from the preceding discussion is of a group of almost stereotypical ethical models that do not correspond in any easy one-to-one fashion with the views and problems of the actual health care policy arena. The priority-setting debate is located in constantly shifting terrain somewhere between the main ethical concerns of deontology, consequentialism and justice. There are many shades of opinion lying upon a number of continua. There are strict deontological health workers just as there are strict welfare utilitarian economists, but between lies a large body of consequentialists who are concerned about equity as well as utility, and who acknowledge the importance of the deontological dimension. The lack of convergence between these theoretical ethical models and the practical models for priority setting contributes to the confusion surrounding the debate.

The most likely groups to promote explicit rationing are those holding consequentialist views; in practice the most active in this field have been health economists. Groups with such ethical principles are not only likely to promote explicit rationing, but also technical methodologies upon which to base this rationing. For example, health economists tend to promote technical methods based on efficiency. Those holding deontological views are the least likely to accept that choices about health care must be made, and thus it follows that they are the most likely to provide opposition to the introduction of explicit priority setting.

The majority of individuals and groups, however, fall between the two extremes of strict deontology and strict utilitarianism, employing a "mix and match" of ethical principles. They have no single underlying ethical model, but choose aspects of the models to suit their own purposes. It is therefore not clear on what ethical basis priority setting will then take place. For pluralistic bargaining this issue may be less important as it is grounded in the hybrid ethical bases of its participants. Inevitably, pluralistic bargaining will be specific to the society in which it is conducted, its time, and to that part of society involved in its process.

What is required is an acknowledgement of ethical complexity, combined with a change in the style and nature of debate about the ethics of priority setting. As Margaret Somerville, a Canadian academic, has argued, the strength of "doing ethics" lies in "making us sensitive to moral diversity, to the pluralism of our society, to the need for respect for others and their values, and, in most cases, to the need for active tolerance".[54] A subtle shift is required in the nature of political discourse, towards the sort of analytical rigour that ethicists commend and away from the intellectually evasive style of much political debate. A wider awareness of the ethical canvas is lacking in many of the discussions about priority setting. Each group is in danger of occupying its own ethical niche unaware of the landscape around. While there are differences in the various perspectives, these have often been exaggerated, especially in public debate, where rhetoric tends to triumph over reason. There is thus the need to acknowledge the value of a multidisciplinary approach to priority setting in health care to avoid the inevitable alternative: conflict.

REFERENCES

1. Gillon R. *Philosphical medical ethics*. John Wiley, Chichester, 1985.
2. Lieban RW. Medical anthropology and the comparative study of ethics. In: Weisz G, ed. *Social science perspectives on medical ethics*. Kluwer Academic, Dordrecht, 1990.
3. Kunstadter P. Medical ethics in cross-cultural and multi-cultural perspectives. *Soc Sci Med* 1980; **148**: 289–96.
4. ten Have H. Ethics and economics in health care: a medical philosopher's view. In: Mooney G, McGuire A, eds. *Medical ethics and economics in health care*. Oxford University Press, Oxford, 1988.
5. Glover J. *Causing death and saving lives*. Penguin, Harmondsworth, 1977.
6. Caplan AL. Can applied ethics be effective in health care and should it

strive to be? In: Caplan AL, ed. *If I were a rich man could I buy a pancreas?* Indiana University Press, Bloomington, 1992.

7. Acton HB. Comte's positivism and the science of society. *Philosophy* 1951; **26**: 291–310.

8. Hoffmaster B. Morality and the social sciences. In: Weisz G, ed. *Social science perspectives on medical ethics*. Kluwer Academic, Dordrecht, 1990.

9. Seedhouse D. *Ethics: the heart of health care*. John Wiley, Chichester, 1988.

10. Young A. Moral conflicts in a psychiatric hospital treating combat related post traumatic stress disorder (PTSD). In: Weisz G, ed. *Social science perspectives on medical ethics*. Kluwer Academic, Dordrecht, 1990.

11. Menzel PT. *Strong medicine*. Oxford University Press, Oxford, 1990.

12. Hamlyn DW. *A history of western philosophy*. Penguin, Harmondsworth, 1987.

13. Kilner JF. *Who lives? Who dies? Ethical criteria in patient selection*. Yale University Press, New Haven, 1990.

14. Winslow GR. *Triage and justice*. University of California Press, Berkeley, 1982.

15. Hadorn DC. Setting health care priorities in Oregon. Cost-effectiveness meets the rule of rescue. *J Am Med Assoc* 1991; **265**(17): 2218–25.

16. Brown A. *Modern political philosophy*. Penguin, Harmondsworth, 1986.

17. Black D. *An anthology of false antitheses*. Nuffield Provincial Hospitals Trust, London, 1984.

18. Rutten FFH. Introduction. In: Mooney G, McGuire A, eds. *Medical ethics and economics in health care*. Oxford University Press, Oxford, 1988.

19. Weale A, ed. *Costs and choice in health care: the ethical dimension*. Kings Fund, London, 1988.

20. Rhodes P. *An outline history of medicine*. Butterworths, London, 1985.

21. Stacey M. The British General Medical Council and medical ethics. In: Weisz G, ed. *Social science perspectives on medical ethics*. Kluwer Academic, Dordrecht, 1990.

22. Proctor R. *Racial hygiene: medicine under the Nazis*. Harvard University Press, Cambridge, MA, 1988.

23. Sohl P. Financing of medical services and medical ethics. In: Mooney G, McGuire A, eds. *Medical ethics and economics in health care*. Oxford University Press, Oxford, 1988.

24. Mooney G, McGuire A. Economics and medical ethics in health care: an economic viewpoint. In: Mooney G, McGuire A, eds. *Medical ethics and economics in health care*. Oxford University Press, Oxford, 1988.

25. Levinsky NG. The doctor's master. *N Engl J Med* 1984; **311**: 1573–5.

26. Faber-Langendoen K. Ethical issues in the allocation and reimbursement of bone marrow transplantation. *Leukemia* 1993; **7**: 1117–21.

27. Doyal L, Wilsher D. Withholding cardiopulmonary resuscitation: proposals for formal guidelines. *BMJ* 1993; **306**: 1593–6.
28. Gillon R. Ethics, economics and general practice. In: Mooney G, McGuire A, eds. *Medical ethics and economics in health care*. Oxford University Press, Oxford, 1988.
29. Lamb D. *Organ transplants and ethics*. Routledge, London, 1990.
30. Neuberger JM. Transplantation for alcoholic liver disease. *BMJ* 1989; **299**: 693–4.
31. Veatch RM. *Case studies in medical ethics*. Harvard University Press, Cambridge, MA, 1977.
32. Rees AM. *TH Marshall's social policy in the twentieth century*. Hutchinson, London, 1985.
33. Mooney G, Drummond MF. What is economics? *BMJ* 1982; **285**: 949–50.
34. Mooney G, Jensen UJ. Changing values and changing policy. In: Jenson UJ, Mooney G, eds. *Changing values in medical and health care decision making*. John Wiley, Chichester, 1990.
35. Mooney G, Gerard K, Donaldson C, Farrar S. *Priority setting in purchasing. Some practical guidelines*. NAHAT, Birmingham, 1992.
36. Culyer AJ. The morality of efficiency in health care – some uncomfortable implications. *Health Econ* 1992; **1**(1): 7–18.
37. Maynard A. Logic in medicine: an economist's perspective. *BMJ* 1987; **295**: 1537–41.
38. Shenkin HA. Rationing of medical care. *Lancet* 1989; **i**: 1392.
39. Ham C. Health care rationing. *BMJ* 1995; **310**: 1483–4.
40. Anon. Doctors won't play the rationing game. *BMA News Rev (Hospital Edn)* 1993; **April**: 8.
41. Green DG. *The new right*. Wheatsheaf, Brighton, 1987.
42. Harris J. *The value of life*. Routledge & Kegan Paul, London, 1985.
43. Hope T, Sprigings D, Crisp R. "Not clinically indicated": patients' interests or resource allocation? *BMJ* 1993; **306**: 379–81.
44. Hare RM. *Moral thinking*. Oxford University Press, Oxford, 1981.
45. Veatch RM. Justice and outcomes research: the ethical limits. *J Clin Ethics* 1993; **4**: 258–61.
46. Rawls J. *A theory of justice*. Oxford University Press, Oxford, 1977.
47. Caplan AL. Introduction. In: Caplan AL, ed. *If I were a rich man could I buy a pancreas?* Indiana University Press, Bloomington, 1992.
48. Doyal L, Gough I. *A theory of human need*. MacMillan, Basingstoke, 1991.
49. Broome J. Fairness versus doing the most good. *Hastings Center Report* 1994; **July–August**: 36–9.
50. Charny MC, Lewis PA, Farrow SC. Choosing who shall not be treated in the NHS. *Soc Sci Med* 1989; **28**: 1331–8.
51. Ashmore M, Mulkay M, Pinch T. *Health and efficiency: a sociology of health*

economics. Open University Press, Milton Keynes, 1989.
52. Moore GE. *Principia ethica*. Cambridge University Press, Cambridge, 1903.
53. Pellegrino ED. *The virtuous physician and the ethics of medicine*. D Reidel, Dordrecht, 1985.
54. Somerville MA. Ethics and clinical practice guidelines. *Can Med Assoc J* 1993; **148**: 1133–7.

PART THREE

Technical Priority Setting and the Equity–Efficiency Conflict

CHAPTER FIVE

JOANNA COAST

Efficiency: The Economic Contribution to Priority Setting

The concept of efficiency is central to the models and techniques proposed by economists. Economists define an efficient outcome as one that maximises the benefit which can be obtained from the available allocation of resources. Efficiency is not about saving money for the NHS, but about increasing the amount of benefit that can be produced from a given level of health care resources. The economic contribution to priority setting is based on the principle of efficiency, although the need to consider other principles such as equity is generally acknowledged by economists.

The purpose of this chapter is to discuss the approaches to the rationing debate developed by economists, the progress that has been made and some of the problems and difficulties encountered. The meaning of efficiency is discussed in some detail before two techniques for priority setting are examined: economic evaluation, and programme budgeting and marginal analysis.

EFFICIENCY AS A BASIS FOR PRIORITY SETTING

The achievement of (greater) efficiency is usually put forward by economists as the main objective of priority setting in health care.

Priority Setting: The Health Care Debate.
Edited by J. Coast, J. Donovan and S. Frankel.   © 1996 John Wiley & Sons Ltd.

Economists separate "efficiency" into different types. The simplest type of efficiency to attain is that of producing a given output at a minimum cost,[1,2] as is used when evaluating interventions which aim to treat the same condition. This type of efficiency is variously known as technical efficiency,[1,2] × efficiency,[3] operational efficiency[4] and cost-effectiveness.[5,6] It will be referred to here as technical efficiency. Unfortunately, achieving or knowing about this type of efficiency is not sufficient for setting priorities.

Those whose aim is to set priorities across health care services must consider a "higher" level of efficiency known as allocative efficiency. This is because priority setting involves not just deciding the most cost-effective way of treating each condition, but deciding which conditions to treat. The theoretical basis behind optimal allocative efficiency is that it should be the state where "it is not possible to make any individual better off without making some other individual worse off" (McGuire et al,[1] p.76). In practice, it is assumed that one state is better than another if those who lose from a change in policy could, theoretically, be compensated by those who gain. The efficiency criterion is thus adapted to one of "ensuring that goods and services are allocated so as to maximise the welfare of the community" (Drummond,[2] p.100). This level of efficiency is also sometimes known as "top-level" or "global" efficiency.[5] It cannot be achieved unless there is also technical efficiency in the production of individual health care services.

While the objective of maximising welfare may seem relatively simple and self-evident, it ignores a number of possible supplementary or alternative objectives. It is the convention in economics to ignore issues concerning equity or just distribution – benefit to society should be maximised on the assumption that there is already a just or satisfactory distribution. The following statement made by Donaldson and Mooney outlines the economic approach to priority setting.

> The aim of priority setting is to ensure that the health benefits resulting from health care are maximised and that the opportunity costs of health care are minimised. (Donaldson and Mooney,[7] p.1529)

There is no part of this statement that allows for the possibility of other objectives in the provision of health care. Economic models are therefore necessarily relatively narrow, although it is frequently stated that distributional aspects should be considered alongside the results obtained through economic techniques. In any case, economic models are most certainly not intended to replace those making decisions. They are intended only to provide additional information to assist those formulating health policy.

It is important to consider precisely what is the definition of "benefit" in the context of efficiency. The most traditional models (welfare economic models[5]) assume that the individuals' satisfaction (or utility) depends upon their consumption of goods or services: thus "benefit" is concerned with the utility obtained from the consumption of these goods and services, and it is this utility which should be maximised. In less traditional models (extra-welfare economic models[5]) it is assumed that satisfaction (or utility) depends in part on things other than the goods and services consumed, for example health: thus "benefit" may depend on health gains, and so some techniques are based on the maximisation of health gain. The interpretation of this concept of "benefit" gives rise to different techniques for priority setting.

If interventions that are perceived to provide the greatest benefit per unit of cost are given priority this will lead to the maximisation of benefit per unit of cost. The perception of greatest benefit will, however, be dependent upon what is perceived to be a benefit and how it is measured and valued. Further, the desire to maximise benefit immediately produces the problem of how to assess benefit using a common measure across different forms of health care – without which the comparison of different types of intervention would be difficult or impossible. The quality-adjusted life-year (QALY) is one response to this difficulty, although money also provides a common measure.

It is also important to consider that "benefit" may accrue not only to the individual receiving the health treatment, but to others – who may benefit purely from knowing that care is being received. Explicit priority setting may therefore influence the total benefit obtained not just through the choices made, but also through the knowledge that some people with need will not receive treatment. This could provide an argument against explicit priority setting.

In the next section the "ideal" technique of economic evaluation will be considered as a means of setting priorities. The chapter will then consider a more pragmatic approach which has been advocated, that of programme budgeting and marginal analysis (PBMA).

ECONOMIC EVALUATION

In economic evaluation, alternative uses of resources are compared by relating the benefits which result from particular options to the associated costs in terms of real resource use.[8] Using the techniques of economic evaluation as a basis for setting priorities requires that priorities are to be set between different programmes, on the basis of the cost of the intervention and its benefit. Such priorities therefore relate to the intervention rather than the individual. This does not, of course, preclude comparing the costs and benefits for the treatment of different severities of a condition as well as different conditions. Indeed it is important that both aspects are considered.

There are three main techniques available for economic evaluation, but they are not all equally useful for the purposes of priority setting. The simplest technique, cost-effectiveness analysis, is not appropriate for setting priorities as it does not provide a common measure of benefit across different forms of health care and hence is able to deal only with questions of technical efficiency. The two methods of economic evaluation that are able to deal with questions of allocative efficiency are cost–benefit analysis and cost–utility analysis. In the first of these benefit is measured in terms of monetary values, and in the second it is measured in terms of utility (usually the QALY).

Although Donaldson and Mooney state that "In an ideal world [there] would be a cost benefit assessment of all treatments at all possible levels of provision and the selection of those that yielded the greatest benefit per pound spent" (Donaldson and Mooney,[7] p.1530), there are problems with cost–benefit analysis which make its use unacceptable to many for the purposes of priority setting. All outcomes in cost–benefit analysis are measured in terms of money and are therefore dependent largely on ability to pay. Because the existing income distribution is unequal (although assumed by economic techniques to be in some way correct/desirable/ acceptable), interventions which are particularly desired or needed by those with higher wealth or income are likely to be more highly valued using this measure. Thus, use of this technique could mean that certain interventions are more likely to be given priority, and therefore, that the setting of priorities is to some extent a function of income and/or wealth. The implicit acceptance of such a value judgement by the use of cost–benefit analysis is at odds with the principles upon which the National Health Service was founded.

Practically, there are also problems with valuing health care benefits in monetary terms as this is an activity with which the public is unfamiliar, in the UK at least. Large sectors of the public also find it unacceptable and may hence be unwilling to participate in such exercises. The difficulty of valuing in monetary terms all the benefits accruing from a health care intervention is a problem specific to the use of cost–benefit analysis, and is one of the main reasons that cost–benefit analysis has tended to be bypassed in the priority-setting debate.

For these reasons cost–benefit analysis will not be discussed further in this section. The remainder of the section will concentrate on cost–utility analysis, which has already been used for the purpose of setting priorities, and is the method of economic evaluation which appears to have most potential for the future.

COST–UTILITY ANALYSIS

The notion of using cost–utility analysis, in particular QALYs, for priority setting in health care is highly controversial. There are both those who strongly advocate its use, arguing that the method is at least as good as the present level of intuitive decision-making,[9-11] and those who disagree with any suggestion that it should be used.[12-14]

Cost–utility analysis uses "utility" as a basis for the measurement of the benefits of health care (for a fuller exposition of the methodology see Drummond, Stoddart and Torrance[8]). Utility can be perceived either as a measure of satisfaction or as a statement of preference. The basis of cost–utility analysis is that changes in cost are compared with changes in (health-related) utility as the chosen measure of benefit. Efficiency occurs when health-related utility is maximised for a given cost, or alternatively, when cost is minimised for given health-related utility.

In its most common current forms, cost–utility analysis only values changes in utility resulting from alterations in health status (i.e. health "output" or health-related utility is taken to be the maximand[5]). Thus, no value is given to parallel changes in utility occurring as a result of information provision or decision-making on the part of others (so-called process utility).[15] Furthermore, the majority of analyses consider only changes in the utility of the patient, and do not take into account changes affecting either the relatives of the patient, or, perhaps more importantly in some cases, the effects of health care on the patient's carer. The implication of using a model which considers only health-related utility is that health improvement of the patient under consideration is the only objective of health care provision.

When the cost- and utility-gained elements of the analysis are combined, a figure for marginal cost per unit of utility gained (or the extra cost per extra unit of utility) can be obtained for each intervention. All other things being equal, those interventions with a low marginal cost per unit of utility gained should receive a greater priority (resource allocation) than those with a higher cost per unit of utility gained, where there are individuals needing both treatments. By always carrying out the most beneficial action with every unit of cost, it is possible to maximise benefit – theoretically at least.

There are a number of different methods available at present for the measurement of health-related utility. The majority of these are of the quality-adjusted life-year (QALY) type, but alternatives to the QALY include the Healthy Year Equivalent (HYE)[16,17] and the saved young life equivalent (SAVE).[18] The QALY has been used in the majority of practical cost–utility analyses that have been conducted to date,[6] and will be the method discussed in the remainder of this section.

The QALY is not a pure utility measure as it considers only one particular characteristic of the individual's utility, i.e. that part of utility concerned with the individual's health status. The QALY is calculated by weighting future life expectancy for the expected quality of life during this time. The maximum value for each future year of life is usually 1: only a year of life during which "perfect health" is experienced is given this value. Death is usually valued at zero. The majority of less than perfect health states fall between zero and one, although some valuations have been obtained which imply that at least some individuals value some health states at less than zero,[19-21] that is, as worse than death.

A number of health status indices have been developed from which QALYs can be formed. These include the Rosser Index[19-21] developed in the UK, the Quality of Well Being Scale[22-24] developed in the USA, and the Health Status Classification Index[8,25] developed in Canada. Other QALYs have been formed from disease-specific indices.[6,26,27] In addition, the EuroQol group has formed a new health status index, from which QALYs may be formed,[28,29] Rosser et al are developing a new measure, the Index of Health-Related Quality of Life,[30] and researchers are exploring the possibility of obtaining utility valuations for the SF36, a US profile measure of health.[31] Each of these indices includes varying numbers of health dimensions. For example, in its original form, the Rosser Index has only two dimensions (disability and distress), whilst the Health Status Classification Index has four dimensions (physical function, role function, social–emotional function and health problem) and the EuroQol has five dimensions (mobility, self-care, usual activities, pain/discomfort, anxiety/depression).

The main index that has been used in the formation of QALYs and which uses UK-obtained valuations, is the Rosser Index.[19,20] The original valuations for this index were derived from 70 respondents, including 10 doctors, 20 nurses, 20 patients and 20 healthy volunteers.[32] The Rosser Index has been criticised in the past for the small number of dimensions it incorporates,[33] as well as for the small number of individuals upon which its valuations are based,[6] and for the selective nature of the respondents. Further valuations for the Rosser Index have, however, been obtained from work in York.[34] Although the Rosser Index has in the past been extensively used in the UK, the EuroQol is more likely to be used in the future.

The usefulness of cost–utility analysis for the purpose of priority setting depends to a large extent on whether the measures used suffer from theoretical or practical problems, and on how acceptable they are perceived to be. Notwithstanding this, there are two possible ways in which cost–utility analysis could be used for the purposes of priority setting. The first is to evaluate all possible options at once, as in Oregon's first attempt at setting priorities[35] (see Chapter 2). The second is to combine results from individual studies into marginal cost per QALY league tables.[6] The problems associated with both approaches are discussed below.

ECONOMIC EVALUATION AS TECHNICAL PRIORITY SETTING

There is little doubt that economic evaluation forms one of the major technical methods for setting priorities, and as such suffers from the associated problems. There are great practical difficulties in acquiring the required large quantities of detailed data: data on all aspects of cost and benefit for numerous different treatments for numerous different health problems. Most of these data are neither routinely available nor easy to generate. Difficulties in attempting to acquire such data for a large-scale exercise (based on cost–utility analysis) across the whole system of health care were experienced in Oregon,[35] (see Chapter 2) and similar problems were faced by the UK's North Western Regional Health Authority when it attempted to allocate regional specialty development funds for 1987/88 on the basis of a cost–utility analysis.[36] In this latter attempt it was only possible to complete cost/QALY calculations for 28% of the 95 bids for specialty funds.[36] Problems in data acquisition may be the greatest hindrance in the use of economic evaluation for priority setting.[37]

The alternative to attempting to set priorities across a number of services in one go, is to use the piecemeal "QALY league table" approach. With this approach, the results of different cost–utility analyses are compared in the form of a league table. The approach, however, has its own set of snares. Studies may be conducted at different times; they may be conducted in different locations; they may be conducted using different quality of life measures which incorporate different values; and they may contain different ranges of costs.[38,39] Each of these factors will reduce the comparability across different items in such a table.

Additional to the problems of data collection are those of implementation. There is no natural link between the lists generated and routine clinical practice (such as might be expected with a bargaining approach in which clinicians are involved). The expectation that such lists will somehow become integrated into clinical practice may therefore be naïve.

ECONOMIC EVALUATION: THE EFFICIENCY BASIS

Cost–utility analysis involves a different concept from that of cost–benefit analysis, at least in its current form of QALYs, because it is concerned with the maximisation of health-related utility rather than utility more generally. There are difficulties, however, in defining "health". The exact concept of efficiency used in cost–utility analysis thus rests on how "health" is defined. There are decisions to be made concerning the dimensions to be included in the QALY measure. They might at a broad level include: disability, distress, pain, ability to fulfil role, social–emotional health, mobility, anxiety/distress, etc. But there are more specific aspects of health, such as relief from urinary symptoms, which might not be reflected in such measures. Should they be included? And who should decide? The dimensions which may be relevant to "health gain" are not self-evident, and it is unlikely, practically, that all possible dimensions could be included. Furthermore, within each dimension, the component health states must be defined. Again this has implications for what is being maximised and thus the type of efficiency that will be achieved.

There is a further decision to be made about who should carry out the valuations involved. This could be any combination of the government, health service, society in general, clinicians, patients and so on. In general, QALY measures have attempted to use societal judgements, although this has not always been the case.

DIFFICULTIES IN ACHIEVING EFFICIENCY THROUGH ECONOMIC EVALUATION

There are substantial theoretical and methodological problems associated with QALYs, and thus cost–utility analysis, which have implications for the technique as a basis for priority setting.

Theoretical Problems

It is not the aim here to give a full critique of the theoretical problems associated with QALYs. (The interested reader is referred elsewhere.[14,15,33,40,41]) It is important, however, to consider the ramifications that such theoretical problems might have for the use of QALYs in priority setting.

The majority of theoretical criticisms of QALYs are directed at the assumptions upon which the methodology is based. Not all the criticisms are applicable to all forms of QALY measurement, because the way in which valuations are obtained varies from one type of QALY to another (see below). The most basic assumptions underlying the QALY methodology, however, are that it is possible to say not only that one health state is better than another, but also how much better it is; that it is possible to equate the prospect of living for Y years in less than full health to the prospect of living for X years in full health, where X is less than Y;[33] and that it is possible to compare utility scores across individuals.

Further assumptions of the QALY procedure include first, that the same ranking of alternatives would occur whether a separate assessment of each period of life was made and then aggregated to produce a total utility, or whether an overall assessment of utility was made;[5] second, that two extra QALYs to individual A are equal to two times one extra QALY to individual A; third, that individuals do not, per se, prefer a less risky outcome to a more risky outcome.[33] These assumptions are not exhaustive, although they include some of the most important and most criticised of the assumptions.

The use of QALYs, and other forms of utility assessment, is dependent on these assumptions reflecting "reality", or at least modelling "reality" in an acceptable fashion. Without rigorous testing of these assumptions it is difficult to determine whether they are realistic, and thus whether a model which incorporates these assumptions should be used for health service planning. However, although the assumptions behind the QALY procedure are important, it is equally important to consider how well the model predicts the choices that would be made by individuals given a similar level of information and thus how closely it predicts the maximisation of health-related utility. As Loomes and McKenzie state:

> In all cases, there should be attempts to compare the choices between various alternatives implied by the stated valuations and QALY scores derived, with decisions made in direct choices between those same alternatives. (Loomes and McKenzie,[33] p.307)

If QALYs accurately predict the way people value health and extra years of life, then the use of QALYs will result in the same choices that informed utility-maximising individuals would make, and would lead to the maximisation of the benefit obtained from health care resources. The acceptability of the strong assumptions used then becomes a less important issue. Alternatively, if QALYs do not accurately predict the ways in which health is valued, it may be necessary to relax or adapt the assumptions, or even to look for alternative measures of health gain or utility.

Methodological Problems

There are a number of methods available for obtaining valuations for incorporation in QALY measures, including the standard gamble, time trade-off, category scaling and magnitude estimation. All involve somewhat hypothetical exercises in which individuals are asked to assign values to particular health states, in some cases directly and in others by more indirect routes. Each of these methods is described briefly below, before the associated problems are examined. Interested readers can find more detailed descriptions of the methods elsewhere.[8,42]

A rating scale generally consists of either a horizontal or vertical line with clearly defined endpoints.[8] The individual is asked to put the most preferred health state at one end of the scale, and the least preferred at the other end. Intermediate health states are then placed on the line so that the order represents the individual's preference ordering, and so that the difference between placements represents the individual's difference in preference for different health states. It is then possible to obtain values for all states on the basis that death is valued at zero, and that perfect health is given the value 1. This method has been used to obtain values for the EuroQol.[28]

The standard gamble is generally considered the "gold standard" in terms of assessing utilities.[8] Individuals are asked to choose between two alternatives. In one the individual will have the certainty of an intermediate health state for n years. In the other the individual will have perfect health for n years with probability p, or will die immediately with probability $(1 - p)$. The value of p is manipulated until the individual is indifferent between the two alternatives. This value, p, is then equivalent to the preference value for the intermediate health state.

The time trade-off technique asks individuals to choose between an intermediate health state lasting for $n1$ years followed immediately by death, and a perfect health state lasting for $n2$ years and followed immediately by death, where $n2$ is less than $n1$.[8] The value of $n2$ is varied until the individual is indifferent between the two alternatives. The value of $n2/n1$ is then equal to the preference value for the intermediate health state.

During magnitude estimation individuals are asked to say how many times better (or worse) it is to experience one state compared with another.[34] It is then possible to scale the answers given, again using zero to represent death and unity to represent perfect health. This method was used to form the original values for the Rosser Index.[19]

The use of utilities as a means of obtaining information about preferences for use in priority setting is somewhat indirect (for information about other methods see Chapter 8). It does not give individuals the opportunity to express directly their preference for one service over another, or to explain why they hold a particular view. An advantage of the method, however, is that it can involve the public without requiring them to have an extensive medical knowledge or an extensive knowledge of the health service. The method may require individuals to make judgements that they find very difficult and is likely to require considerable research time. There are particular difficulties posed by the interpersonal comparison of individual utilities. Economists are divided on the issue of interpersonal comparison of utility. While classical expected utility theory rejects the notion that it is scientifically meaningful to compare individual preferences,[15,43,44] a number of economists insist that comparison of preferences is essential, and that, in any case, such comparisons are common practice in social decision-making.[45-47] The question of the comparability of preferences is important because it largely determines whether or not individual utilities can be aggregated to provide a collective social preference. Torrance et al argue that comparison of individual preferences is valid, and that it is, then, important to consider how such comparisons should be made.[47] [Torrance et al choose to use two clearly defined outcomes as "anchor points" (healthy life and immediate death), and then set the difference in utility between these two points equal across individuals. The arithmetic mean is then used to aggregate preferences.[47] The arithmetic mean is also recommended by Harsanyi.[45,46]]

There are a number of problems common to all survey procedures of this type which may affect the utility valuations obtained: there may be difficulties concerning the extent to which survey procedures are perceived to be real by those participating in the survey;[41] the ways in which the different alternatives are described can affect the values individuals give them;[48] and framing effects may occur, that is, where individuals respond with different valuations for the *same* question when it is shown in a positive light compared with when it is shown in a negative light.[33,49]

Problems specific to QALYs include people being asked to value health states against death when no one knows what death will be like,[41] and that valuations may creep towards 1 as health states deteriorate naturally with age.[33] In addition to these problems, different methods of eliciting values have been shown to lead to notable differences in the indices obtained.[33] Unfortunately, even using the same method of deriving values may not always lead to the same indices, for example, the standard gamble (the "gold standard") has shown this tendency. This is a problem of internal consistency, where starting with different pairs of probabilities generates different sets of utilities.[33,50]

Each of these methodological problems will impact on the ability of economic evaluation to provide information about efficiency for use in priority setting.

EQUITY AND ECONOMIC EVALUATION

Economic evaluation is based almost exclusively on the notion of efficiency. The aim is to maximise, regardless of the subsequent distributional effects. As a result there has been extensive discussion of the equity implications of QALYs. They have frequently been referred to as ageist and criticised on this basis.[51,52] QALYs are currently weighted on an equal basis for all individuals, but they could alternatively be weighted on the basis of particular variables such as age, gender, number of children, occupation, risk-bearing activities, etc.[34,53] In this way equity objectives as well as efficiency objectives could be inbuilt within the QALY measure used and thus within the subsequent economic evaluation.

CONCLUSION: ECONOMIC EVALUATION

Choices between different forms of economic evaluation as methodologies for priority setting do not just depend on the relative merits of the two techniques. They also depend fundamentally on what the objectives of the NHS are perceived to be. If the primary objective is assumed to be to improve the health of the population then it is unlikely that cost–benefit analysis can be considered appropriate. This is because the assumption used by cost–benefit analysis is that it is appropriate to base valuations of health benefit on willingness (and therefore ability) to pay.

If cost–benefit analysis cannot assist in priority setting, this leaves cost–utility analysis. Although there appears to be great potential for using this technique for priority setting,[7] there are difficulties in acquiring valid, reliable utility values which correspond to economic theory. A further problem, with QALYs at least, is that health may not be the only output of health care which is valued by society. Mooney and colleagues have identified a number of other potential benefits which may also be important, including reassurance and the ability to participate in decision-making.[4]

Should all the theoretical and methodological problems associated with cost–utility analysis be overcome, however, it is unlikely that it would, in isolation, make a sound basis for priority setting across the entire set of options on which health services could spend their money. This is because of one of the major problems associated with technical methods of priority setting: it is unlikely that sufficient data will ever be generated to cover the wide variety of possible health problems and possible reactions to those health problems. It may be that economic evaluation is useful when applied in a piecemeal manner, to a restricted set of options, and in conjunction with other methods so as to take account of objectives other than maximising health gain. This is far from the "holy grail" of an explicit set of priorities for health care, however, and the use of so-called QALY league tables has its own set of difficulties,[4,39,54] not least of which is the quality of many of the studies conducted to date.[6]

PROGRAMME BUDGETING AND MARGINAL ANALYSIS

Given that many economists feel that economic evaluation would, in an ideal world, be the preferred method of priority setting, but that the data requirements of such an approach are vast, "a more pragmatic" alternative has been suggested.[7] This is generally referred to as programme budgeting and marginal analysis (PBMA).[4]

Although the specific approach of PBMA has only been recently promoted as a means of setting priorities in health care, it has as its predecessors the US Planning-Programming-Budgeting System (PPBS) and, in the UK, the Public Expenditure Survey.[52,55,56] The application of programme budgeting to health care has also been advocated in the past.[57,58] Although many governments introduced programme budgeting in its heyday during the 1960s and 1970s the system is generally regarded as having failed in its most ambitious forms.[55,59] There are, however, organisations, such as local authorities in Australia, [59] who are still experimenting with programme budgeting.

The main advocates of PBMA as a means of deciding on priorities for health care in the UK are Donaldson and Mooney.[4,7] These authors state that health authorities must decide which programmes are relevant to the strategy of the health authority in terms of disease groups, client groups or specialties.[7] The chosen programmes (between 10 and 20 are thought to be a manageable number[4]), it is recommended, should have some degree of homogeneity of output, and it must be possible to at least approximate the costs of activities within the programme.[7] Each programme should then be inspected to see whether reallocations within the programme could generate an overall increase in benefits, i.e. undertaking economic evaluation for the particular marginal changes identified. The ultimate stage of PBMA would then be to perform this procedure across the programmes. Practical examples of PBMA in the last few years have tended to confine themselves to analysis within programmes rather than attempting to consider allocation across programmes.[60]

The proposed strategy is intended as a practical response to the difficulties of applying economic evaluation in a detailed manner. The method advocated by Donaldson and Mooney for making decisions *within programmes* is as follows:

(a) decide which treatments are so valuable or simply have to be provided that it would be a waste of time analysing them;
(b) of the remainder, start by assessing which areas are most open to change;
(c) for each existing programme in turn, divide it into subprogrammes and then ask what the effect would be (if possible in terms of both workload and health) of reducing spending by £100,000 and of increasing it by £100,000. Judgements could then be made on whether some subprogrammes could be cut to allow other subprogrammes to get extra funding so that there would be more benefits in total. (Donaldson and Mooney,[7] p.1530)

Within part (c) above, the terminology has become that of developing "wish" (or incremental wish) lists for those sub-programmes for which there are desirable increases in services, and "death" (or decremental wish) lists for those programmes which could potentially be reduced in scale.[59]

Although PBMA has been advocated only relatively recently, there have already been a number of practical applications of the technique (see for example the work by Brambleby,[61] Cohen,[62]

Donaldson and Farrar,[63] Madden et al,[64] and Twaddle and colleagues[59,65]).

PBMA: TECHNICAL PRIORITY SETTING WITH ELEMENTS OF BARGAINING?

The aim of Donaldson and Mooney in suggesting the approach of PBMA was to find a method of economic evaluation for which the data requirements were less stringent than in more formal evaluations. The difficulties in acquiring large amounts of data are a familiar problem for the majority of technical rationing schemes, and are rehearsed above in relation to economic evaluation. Donaldson and Mooney have achieved a less data-intensive approach by introducing elements of pluralistic bargaining into an otherwise technical priority-setting scheme. This combination of the two approaches opens up a number of interesting issues, but to what extent does the approach solve the problems of data acquisition?

Although PBMA limits the number of alternatives to be studied, and thus the amount of data that needs to be acquired, it does not assist in the acquisition of good quality data for those alternatives which are incorporated. At the subprogramme level, neither the costs nor the benefits of the alternatives under consideration are likely to be known with any degree of certainty, apart, perhaps, from conditions which have recently been the subject of research. It is possible that the results obtained through this method could become subject to similar objections to those which were aimed at the Oregon project, that the data were too poor to make such decisions.[66-70] Although the use of marginal costs is advocated, in very many cases such costs are just not available without detailed (and hence costly and time-consuming) empirical work. Judgements of benefit may also be very subjective; for example, Twaddle and Walker found that it was necessary to make assumptions about changes in outcome rather than acquiring evidence.[65]

The use of pluralistic bargaining as a means of identifying incremental and decremental wish lists may, from an economic viewpoint, be a theoretical disadvantage. There is no theoretical basis for the use of such lists, and, from the viewpoint of a technical rationing scheme, other means of identifying margins which are less reliant on the subjective opinion of individuals who will inevitably have their own areas of self-interest, could potentially be more theoretically sound. For example, there has been extensive work on medical practice variations (see for example Andersen and Mooney[71]) which could provide a means of identifying margins where change may be appropriate. This illustrates the conflict between technical and political bases for rationing: what may be a disadvantage from the viewpoint of a technical rationing scheme is likely to be an advantage from the perspective of pluralistic bargaining. In particular, the use of bargaining groups to assist in these decisions may make the implementation of subsequent policies much more likely.

The incorporation of elements of bargaining in this technical rationing scheme highlights the issue of who should be involved in the aspects of bargaining. Decisions about who should be involved in the PBMA process may lead to considerable differences in the resulting decisions, with those making the choices in a position heavily to influence the services which comprise the "wish" and "death" lists. The only guidance provided about who should be involved is that from Mooney and colleagues who state that they should be "people well placed to form judgements about the impact of various policy changes on the programme" (Mooney et al,[4] p.19). Where the membership of the group is entirely composed of clinicians and purchasers, such as in the work by Twaddle,[59,65] it may be difficult to see how the technique is an advance over other means of making decisions. Practical experience has shown, however, that incorporating others into the group can also prove to be difficult. Cohen states, with reference to two previous attempts to use PBMA, that there have been difficulties in selecting appropriately representative working groups to conduct the exercises.[62,64] Over-representation of any one group, with its associated vested interests, may enable it to monopolise the exercise. This is a particular danger where some groups are inevitably both more knowledgeable and more articulate than others, with clinicians inevitably falling into this category.[72]

PBMA: EFFICIENCY AND EQUITY

A basic problem with PBMA as a technique, as opposed to a means of pluralistic bargaining, is the difficulty in identifying what precisely is to be maximised. The ideal would be to maximise either utility or health-related utility but, as for economic evaluation, good quality data relating to either of these are unlikely to be available. Madden et al conclude that the consequence of this lack of good quality data is that (in the short term) the subjective judgement of local purchasers about what is "better" should be used.[64] Donaldson feels that, at best, exercises will involve merely a description of the possible outcomes of each of the assessed options.[73] In the absence of outcome data, the only other alternative is the use of intermediate outputs such as admissions, bed-days or consultant episodes. However, attempting to maximise any of these intermediate outputs could have dangerous consequences for the real outcomes of care (for example, maximising number of consultant episodes might imply discharging individuals too early; maximising admissions could imply taking less severely ill patients, who require a shorter stay, in preference to the more severely ill). How well PBMA is therefore able to approximate the results of the more formal methods of economic evaluation may therefore be questionable.

Although equity is not explicitly considered in PBMA, it may implicitly affect the results of the analysis. This may be particularly so if potentially efficient but inequitable alternatives are rejected by the decision-making group before these alternatives get as far as the "wish list", or if the judgement of purchasers about what is "better" is the basis for assessing outcome. Madden and colleagues state their concern that the approach of PBMA says nothing about equity explicitly. They conclude that, pragmatically, the only way to proceed is to concentrate on efficiency during the PBMA exercise and consider equity as a separate issue at the end of this exercise.[64]

CONCLUSION: PROGRAMME BUDGETING

PBMA is based on the more formal methods of economic evaluation, but lacks their precision. Donaldson and Mooney aim to offer a pragmatic approach in terms of the economic evaluation of services leading to priority setting. They have identified the constraints in obtaining data for full economic evaluations, and have offered a solution which will at least approximate the best allocation of resources for any programme.[7] Their message is that it is preferable to use a less than perfect measure which is based on the correct framework than an accurate measure based on the wrong method, (where the wrong method is most usually described as that of total needs assessment, described in Chapter 6).[4]

There is a question, however, as to how much the scheme is one of technical rationing based on an efficiency principle and how much it is one of pluralistic bargaining. In practice, the PBMA approach could work quite differently in different localities, leaning perhaps one way or the other, and depending in large part upon the availability of data for the particular programmes under consideration. Without good measures of and/or reasonable evidence about the costs and benefits of each intervention in the programme area, PBMA may well become an exercise in pluralistic bargaining, with resultant priorities strongly affected by the membership of the group and their decisions about what should be "wishes" and what should be "deaths". Some may therefore argue that, from the viewpoint of efficiency, the framework is not the right one. For example, Bevan has made the following observation concerning programme budgeting as applied in the US PPBS and the UK PES

> Systems thinking in that form . . . does not rule out compromises which are inappropriate but which satisfy vested interests. (Bevan, 1983,[55] p.737)

A further real disadvantage of pursuing the PBMA route to priority setting is that it does not, in itself, provide any real impetus for improvements in the amount or quality of data collected. Despite these problems with PBMA, however, it almost certainly offers a more practical way forward than the notion of large-scale exercises based upon cost–utility analysis. It is much more closely grounded in the process by which health care decisions are made and so avoids considering choices which, for political or other reasons, may be completely impractical (and hence wasting resources).

This link with the process of decision-making may also make implementation of the results much more likely than with more distant exercises.

CONCLUSION

This chapter has explained the efficiency-based priority-setting techniques of economic evaluation and PBMA. Both are examples of technical rationing schemes, although PBMA incorporates significant elements of a pluralistic bargaining approach. The application of an efficiency principle as the basis for priority setting implies that the resources will be allocated in such a way that the maximum benefit will be obtained from the resources available, although the precise definition of benefit may vary. Concessions to equity are, however, implicit in these approaches: even in the emphasis that is usually added that economic techniques do not make decisions, but are there only to assist in the formulation of policy.

In Oregon, the Netherlands and New Zealand, some cautious support has been given to the use of economic methods for priority setting. For example, in the Netherlands, where the aim is to set a basic package of care, efficiency forms part of the framework for priority setting: it has been stated that "The Committee feels that limits may, however, be set when the costs are high and the chances of benefit very small" (*Choices in health care*,[74] p.67). The Core Services Committee in New Zealand has also decided that "value for money" must be taken into account in deciding upon core services – but has explicitly concluded that QALYs "cannot currently give us fair answers about which services should be publicly funded".[75]

Up to the early 1990s, practical attempts to set priorities using economic methods concentrated mainly on the use of cost–utility analysis. In Oregon, the first attempt at setting priorities was carried out using an analysis based on cost–utility,[35] although this was later abandoned for a number of reasons, including the poor quality of the data incorporated into the analysis[66-70] (see Chapter 2). Some health authorities in the UK have also attempted to use this methodology.[40,76] For example, the North Western Regional Health Authority in the UK attempted to allocate regional specialty development funds for 1987/88 on this basis.[36] This attempt failed mainly as a result of the lack of necessary data, but also because substantial reservations about the QALY methodology were expressed by both clinicians and representatives of the public and of patients.[36] Cost–utility analysis has also been used to set priorities among waiting list conditions in general surgery.[77] More recently, however, PBMA has gained in ascendancy. A number of attempts have been made to use this approach and incorporate it into purchasing strategies,[59,61,62,64,73] and to date it has appeared relatively successful.

Economic methods are not intended to provide technological fixes to what are essentially complex decisions, but instead should inform and clarify the decision-making process. Although some cautious support has been given to the principle of efficiency and the use of economic methods for setting priorities, economics cannot solve the problems of rationing. It does, however, provide a basis for thinking about the problem.

REFERENCES

1. McGuire A, Henderson J, Mooney G. *The economics of health care. An introductory text.* Routledge & Kegan Paul, London, 1988.
2. Drummond MF. Output measurement for resource-allocation decisions in health care. In: McGuire A, Fenn P, Mayhew K, eds. *Providing health care: the economics of alternative systems of finance and delivery.* Oxford University Press, Oxford, 1991: 99–119.
3. Mooney GH. *Economics, medicine and health care.* Harvester Wheatsheaf, London, 1986.
4. Mooney G, Gerard K, Donaldson C, Farrar S. *Priority setting in purchasing. Some practical guidelines.* NAHAT, Birmingham, 1992.
5. Culyer AJ. The normative economics of health care finance and provision. In: McGuire A, Fenn P, Mayhew K, eds. *Providing health care: the economics of alternative systems of finance and delivery.* Oxford University Press, Oxford, 1991: 65–99.
6. Gerard K. Cost–utility in practice: a policy maker's guide to the state of the art. *Health Policy* 1992; **21**: 249–79.
7. Donaldson C, Mooney G. Needs assessment, priority setting, and contracts for health care: an economic view. *BMJ* 1991; **303**: 1529–30.

8. Drummond MF, Stoddart GL, Torrance GW. *Methods for the economic evaluation of health care programmes.* Oxford University Press, Oxford, 1987.
9. Williams A. How should NHS priorities be determined? *Hospital Update* 1987; **April**: 261–341.
10. Richardson J, Cook J. Cost utility analysis: "new directions" in setting health care priorities. *Aust Health Rev* 1992; **15**(2): 145–54.
11. Walker P. Are QALYs going to be useful to me as a purchaser of health services? In: Hopkins A, ed. *Measures of the quality of life.* Royal College of Physicians, London, 1992: 53–9.
12. Honigsbaum F. *Who shall live? Who shall die? – Oregon's health financing proposals.* King's Fund College, London, 1991.
13. Harris J. QALYfying the value of life. *J Med Ethics* 1987; **13**: 117–23.
14. Carr-Hill RA. Allocating resources to health care: is the QALY (quality adjusted life year) a technical solution to a political problem? *Int J Health Services* 1991; **21**(2): 351–63.
15. Mooney G, Olsen JA. QALYs: where next? In: McGuire A, Fenn P, Mayhew K, eds. *Providing health care: the economics of alternative systems of finance and delivery.* Oxford University Press, Oxford, 1991: 120–40.
16. Mehrez A, Gafni A. Quality-adjusted life years, utility theory, and healthy-years equivalents. *Med Decis Making* 1989; **9**: 142–9.
17. Culyer AJ, Wagstaff A. *QALYs versus HYEs. A theoretical exposition.* Centre for Health Economics, York, 1992.
18. Nord E. An alternative to QALYs: the saved young life equivalent (SAVE). *BMJ* 1992; **305**: 875–7.
19. Rosser R, Kind P. A scale of valuations of states of illness: is there a social consensus? *Int J Epidemiol* 1978; **7**(4): 347–58.
20. Kind P, Rosser R, Williams A. Valuation of quality of life: some psychometric evidence. In: Jones-Lee MW, ed. *The value of life and safety.* North-Holland Publishing Company, Amsterdam, 1982: 159–70.
21. Gudex C, Kind P. *The QALY toolkit.* Centre for Health Economics, York, 1988.
22. Kaplan RM, Anderson JP. The quality of well-being scale: rationale for a single quality of life index. In: Walker SR, Rosser RM, eds. *Quality of life: assessment and application.* MTP Press, Lancaster, 1988: 51–77.
23. Kaplan RM, Anderson JP. The General Health Policy Model: an integrated approach. In: Spilker B, ed. *Quality of life assessments in clinical trials.* Raven Press, New York, 1990: 131–49.
24. Kaplan RM, Bush JW. Health-related quality of life measurement for evaluation research and policy analysis. *Health Psychol* 1981; **1**: 61–80.
25. Boyle MH, Torrance GW, Sinclair JC, Horwood SP. Economic evaluation of neonatal intensive care of very-low-birth-weight infants.

N Engl J Med 1983; **308**: 1330–7.

26. Barry MJ, Mulley AG, Fowler FJ, Wennberg JW. Watchful waiting vs immediate transurethral resection for symptomatic prostatism. The importance of patients' preferences. *J Am Med Assoc* 1988; **259**(20): 3010–17.

27. Woodward R, Boyarsky S, Barnett H. Discounting surgical benefits. Enucleation versus resection of the prostate. *J Med Systems* 1983; **7**(6): 481–93.

28. The EuroQol Group. EuroQol© – a new facility for the measurement of health-related quality of life. *Health Policy* 1990; **16**(3): 199–208.

29. Carr-Hill R. A good measure for Eurohealth? *Health Service J* 1991; **18 July**: 24–5.

30. Rosser R, Cottee M, Rabin R, Selai C. Index of health-related quality of life. In: Hopkins A, ed. *Measures of the quality of life*. Royal College of Physicians, London, 1992: 81–9.

31. Williams A. Measuring functioning and well-being. The Medical Outcomes Study approach, Anita L. Stewart and John E. Ware, Jr., Editors. Duke University Press, Durham and London, 1992. No of pages: 449. ISBN 0-8223-1212-3. [book review]. *Health Econ* 1992; **1**(4): 255–8.

32. Gudex C. *QALYs and their use by the health service*. Centre for Health Economics, York, 1986.

33. Loomes G, McKenzie L. The use of QALYs in health care decision making. *Soc Sci Med* 1989; **28**(4): 299–308.

34. Williams A, Kind P. The present state of play about QALYs. In: Hopkins A, ed. *Measures of the quality of life*. Royal College of Physicians, London, 1992: 21–34.

35. Oregon Health Services Commission. *Prioritization of Health Services. A report to the Governor and Legislature*. Oregon Health Services Commission, 1991.

36. Allen D, Lee RH, Lowson K. The use of QALYs in health service planning. *Int J Health Planning Management* 1989; **4**: 261–73.

37. Coast J. Developing the QALY concept. Exploring the problems of data acquisition. *PharmacoEconomics* 1993; **4**(4): 240–6.

38. Gerard K, Mooney G. *QALY League Tables: three points for concern – goal difference counts*. Health Economics Research Unit, Aberdeen, 1992.

39. Mason J, Drummond M, Torrance G. Some guidelines on the use of cost effectiveness league tables. *BMJ* 1993; **306**: 570–2.

40. Spiegelhalter DJ, Gore SM, Fitzpatrick R, Fletcher AE, Jones DR, Cox DR. Quality of life measures in health care. III: resource allocation. *BMJ* 1992; **305**: 1205–9.

41. Carr-Hill RA. Assumptions of the QALY procedure. *Soc Sci Med* 1989;

28; 469–77.

42. Torrance GW. Measurement of health state utilities for economic appraisal: a review. *J Health Econ* 1986; **5**: 1–30.

43. Mansfield E. Microeconomics. Theory and applications. In: *Welfare Economics*. 5th ed. W W Norton and Company, New York, 1985: 458–88.

44. Hadorn DC. The role of public values in setting health care priorities. *Soc Sci Med* 1991; **32**(7): 773–81.

45. Harsanyi JC. Nonlinear social welfare functions. Do welfare economists have a special exemption from Bayesian rationality? *Theory and Decision* 1975; **6**: 311–32.

46. Harsanyi JC. Cardinal welfare, individualistic ethics, and interpersonal comparisons of utility. *J Pol Econ* 1955; **63**: 309–21.

47. Torrance GW, Boyle MH, Horwood SP. Application of multi-attribute utility theory to measure social preferences for health states. *Operations Res* 1982; **30**(6): 1043–69.

48. Llewellyn-Thomas H, Sutherland HJ, Tibshirani R, Ciampi A, Till JE, Boyd NF. Describing health states: methodologic issues in obtaining values for health states. *Med Care* 1984; **22**(6): 543–52.

49. McNeil BJ, Pauker SG, Sox HC, Tversky A. On the elicitation of preferences for alternative therapies. *N Engl J Med* 1982; **306**(21): 1259–62.

50. Llewellyn-Thomas H, Sutherland HJ, Tibshirani R, Ciampi A, Till JE, Boyd NF. The measurement of patients' values in medicine. *Med Decis Making* 1982; **5**(4): 449–62.

51. Smith A, Maynard A, Grimley Evans J, Harris J. The ethics of resource allocation. Proceedings of a symposium held at the University of Manchester during the 33rd Annual Scientific Meeting of the Society for Social Medicine, September 1989. *J Epid Commun Health* 1990; **44**: 187–90.

52. Wildavsky A. The political economy of efficiency: cost benefit analysis, systems analysis and program budgeting. *Public Admin Rev* 1966; **December**: 292–310.

53. Williams A. Applications in management. In: Teeling-Smith G, ed. *Measuring health: a practical approach*. John Wiley, Chichester, 1988: 225–43.

54. Drummond M, Torrance G, Mason J. Cost-effectiveness league tables: more harm than good? *Soc Sci Med* 1993; **37**(1): 33–40.

55. Bevan RG. The systems approach in Government? Two case studies of programme budgeting. *J Operational Res Soc* 1983; **34**(8): 729–38.

56. Wildavsky A. Rescuing policy analysis from PPBS. *Public Admin Rev* 1969; **March/April**: 189–201.

57. Mooney GH. Programme budgeting in an area health board. *Hosp*

Health Serv Rev 1977; **November**: 379–84.

58. Mooney G. Programme budgeting: an aid to planning and priority setting in health care. *Effective Health Care* 1984; **2**(2): 65–8.

59. Twaddle S, McIlwaine G, Miller A. *Improving gynaecology services within existing resources. A programme budgeting and marginal analysis approach.* Scottish Needs Assessment Programme, Glasgow, 1994.

60. Craig N, Parkin D, Gerard K. Clearing the fog on the Tyne: programme budgeting in Newcastle and North Tyneside Health Authority. *Health Policy* 1995; **33**(2): 127–45.

61. Brambleby P. A survivor's guide to programme budgeting. *Health Policy* 1995; **33**(2): 161–8.

62. Cohen D. Marginal analysis in practice: an alternative to needs assessment for contracting health care. *BMJ* 1994; **309**: 781–4.

63. Donaldson C, Farrar S. Needs assessment: developing an economic approach. *Health Policy* 1993; **25**: 95–108.

64. Madden L, Hussey R, Mooney G, Church E. Public health and economics in tandem: programme budgeting, marginal analysis and priority setting in practice. *Health Policy* 1995; **33**(2): 161–8.

65. Twaddle S, Walker A. Programme budgeting and marginal analysis: application within programmes to assist purchasing in Greater Glasgow Health Board. *Health Policy* 1995; **33**(2): 91–105.

66. Bowling A. Setting priorities in health: the Oregon experiment (part 2). *Nursing Stand* 1992; **6**(38): 28–30.

67. Eddy DM. What's going on in Oregon? *J Am Med Assoc* 1991; **266**(3): 417–20.

68. McBride G. Rationing health care in Oregon. *BMJ* 1990; **301**: 355–6.

69. Nelson RM, Drought T. Justice and the moral acceptability of rationing medical care: the Oregon experiment. *J Med Philos* 1992; **17**: 97–117.

70. Kaplan RM. A quality-of-life approach to health resource allocation. In: Strosberg MA, Weiner JM, Baker R, Fein A, eds. *Rationing America's medical care: the Oregon plan and beyond.* The Brookings Institution, Washington, DC, 1992: 60–77.

71. Andersen TG, Mooney G. *The challenges of medical practice variations.* Macmillan, Basingstoke, 1990.

72. Cohen DR. Messages from Mid Glamorgan: a multi-programme experiment with marginal analysis. *Health Policy* 1995; **33**(2): 147–55.

73. Donaldson C. Economics, public health and health care purchasing: reinventing the wheel. *Health Policy* 1995; **33**(2): 79

74. Government Committee on Choices in Health Care. *Choices in health care.* Ministry of Welfare, Health and Cultural Affairs, Rijswijk, 1992.

75. National Advisory Committee on Core Health and Disability Support Services. *The best of health 2. How we decide on the health and disability*

support services we value most. National Advisory Committee on Core Health and Disability Support Services, Wellington, 1994.
76. Bowling A. Setting priorities in health: the Oregon experiment (part 1). *Nursing Stand* 1992; **6**(37): 29–32.
77. Gudex C, Williams A, Jourdan M et al. Prioritising waiting lists. *Health Trends* 1990; **22**(3): 103–8.

CHAPTER SIX

JOANNA COAST, GWYN BEVAN AND
STEPHEN FRANKEL

An Equitable Basis for Priority Setting?

EQUITY AS A BASIS FOR PRIORITY SETTING

The aim of this chapter is to discuss methods of rationing which have a claim to be equitable in some way. Principles of equity are broadly concerned with the issue of distribution: in terms of priority setting in health care, therefore, the concern is with who will receive the available health care resources. Theories of justice, such as that developed by Rawls (see Chapter 4), inform the discussion of equity, but there has been relatively little development of practical applications for use in priority setting, compared with developments in the area of efficiency (see Chapter 5).

Contributions to this area come from a number of different disciplinary bases. In part this is because equity is a complex concept, with different answers to the question of "what is equitable?" forming conflicting bases for setting priorities. For example, the economist Gavin Mooney has suggested seven alternative definitions of equity.[1] Four of these definitions are based on need and the remainder comprise equal expenditure per capita, equal inputs per capita and equal health. Although equity principles may appeal to need (which in itself may be defined in different ways) they may also appeal to fairness, to age, or to random

Priority Setting: The Health Care Debate.
Edited by J. Coast, J. Donovan and S. Frankel.   © 1996 John Wiley & Sons Ltd.

allocation. Conflicts between those from different disciplinary bases, with their different objectives, have resulted in considerable confusion in this area. Confusion arises not only from interdisciplinary cross-fire, however, but also from unresolved problems within the different disciplines.

There are two broad ambitions that could be pursued by an "equitable" basis for setting priorities for the available health care resources. The first would be to attempt, explicitly via priority setting, to redress the whole issue of current inequalities in health. In practice this would mean attempting to allocate health care resources to those social groups with poorer health status, in order to redress inequalities caused through other facets of society and through shortcomings in other areas of social policy. The second, lesser, ambition would be to focus merely on providing an equitable basis for the distribution of health care resources, without particular regard to redressing those inequalities caused via other aspects of society. In the latter case the aim would be, as part of a policy of explicit priority setting, to meet the claim on health care resources in an equitable manner.

Whatever priority is accorded to redressing inequalities in health, there is no doubt that these inequalities exist in Britain.[2,3] The debate over inequalities of health is concerned largely with the distribution of health, rather than the distribution of health care. Major determinants of health and illness are the social and physical environments experienced by individuals throughout the life course. Health care too can now have a major impact, positive and negative, on health. This could lead to an argument for greater investment in programmes for those forms of morbidity and mortality which would have the implicit consequence of redressing inequalities. But what this position ignores is the uncertain relationship between particular forms of morbidity and the benefits that may or may not follow from medical interest in them. There are general arguments for increasing the quality of housing, for enhancing economic security, for improving nutrition and for other such general measures that may relate in a general way to health. But in relation to specific health care interventions, the question of effectiveness is central. There can be little merit in advocating major health care interventions in areas where the benefit of treatment is questionable.

It would be impossible in this chapter to discuss comprehensively all the potential applications of equity as bases for priority setting in health care. Instead the chapter focuses on two distinctive, and controversial, contributions to the health care priority-setting debate. Although both contributions are primarily concerned with meeting equitably the claim on health care resources, rather than explicitly aiming to redress current inequalities in health, they differ in other ways. First, the two suggestions have come primarily from different disciplines, epidemiology and philosophy. Second, the two suggestions differ in that one is concerned with setting priorities between the treatment of different conditions, whereas the other is concerned with setting priorities on the basis of personal characteristics.

The first suggestion is to set priorities on the basis of providing equal access to care for those in equal need. This is the main epidemiological contribution to priority setting. For the UK, rationing by need provides the main basis for the current implicit rationing. As an explicit means of setting priorities it is also more likely to be acceptable than other principles (such as efficiency or age-based rationing) and is hence an important area for discussion. As a basis for priority setting it has, however, been heavily criticised by some economists. The other suggestion to be discussed, put forward by some philosophers, is that rationing should be based upon age. Under certain circumstances, it has been claimed, such rationing would provide a just means of allocating health care resources. These controversial suggestions have tended to be made primarily in the USA. Each of these alternatives will be discussed in turn.

EQUITY AND NEED

THE EPIDEMIOLOGICAL BASIS FOR NEEDS-BASED RATIONING

Traditional epidemiology is concerned with examining the distribution and determinants of disease. Modern epidemiology has extended its remit to include assessment of the effectiveness of health care interventions. This outline by Matthew[4] sets out the basic position:

> A need for medical care exists when an individual has an illness or disability for which there is an effective and acceptable treatment or cure. It can be defined either in terms of the type of illness or disability causing the need or of the treatment or facilities for treatment required to meet it. A demand for care exists when an individual considers that he has a need and wishes to receive care. Utilisation occurs when an individual actually receives care. Need is not necessarily expressed as demand, and demand is not necessarily followed by utilisation, while, on the other hand, there can be demand and utilisation without real underlying need for the particular service. (Matthews,[4] 1971)

This distinction between need, demand and utilisation, as well as the concern with effectiveness and acceptability, has become intrinsic to any formulation of the health care system. The setting of priorities is not, however, included in this formulation, and, indeed, is not a question that has traditionally been considered by epidemiologists. Just as an account of topography cannot determine the purpose of a journey, portrayals of patterns of disease and health service use offered by epidemiology have, in themselves, no normative value. Determining priorities involves the consideration of what ought to be, rather than what is. While traditional epidemiology offers an account of what to choose between, it does not offer grounds for the choice. It has tended to concern itself with the technical question of assessing need rather than the judgemental question of determining priorities.[5] Despite this, one means of setting priorities equitably has been perceived as being through the assessment of need.

Information about need may additionally inform the extent to which priority setting is required. A very different approach to priority setting would be required where available funding could finance the treatment of 90% of patients with need compared with the situation where only 10% of patients with need could be funded. Central to both the discussion about how priorities should be set and the extent of rationing required, however, is the way in which need is defined. This issue is considered prior to discussion of the potential for setting priorities on the basis of need.

Definitions of Need for Priority Setting

An immediate difficulty is produced by the mandate to assess need in relation to health care service provision: how should need be defined? Need is a complex concept, with many different definitions provided.[6,7] For example, Bradshaw elucidated four types of need: normative need – a desirable standard laid down by experts or professionals; felt need – the wants a population has; expressed need – wants turned into demands; and comparative need – a measure of needs related to the population characteristics of a particular area.[8]

In terms of setting priorities in health care, however, there is one particularly crucial distinction that must be made. This is the difference between defining need as the burden of disease and defining need as capacity to benefit. Need as burden of disease incorporates notions of the severity of the patient's illness and the extent to which this illness exists in the population. It does not, however, include the concept of whether a patient could potentially derive benefit from the provision of treatment. Thus, this definition relates to the need for health. *Health needs* represent the distribution of particular forms of morbidity, as well as the distribution of those environmental, social and economic variables that influence health and illness. Health needs thus offer a comprehensive reflection of the wider environment within which health services function; they broadly reflect the distribution of neediness, but may not distinguish between remediable and irremediable morbidity, and so have an uncertain relationship with health services planning. Nevertheless the assessment of the need for health has a place in broad policy choices, and historically has supplied one basis for resource allocation in the National Health Service (NHS). (For example, see the discussion of RAWP below.)

An alternative definition relates need to capacity to benefit. It incorporates notions of the extent to which patients are able to benefit from the provision of health care. Although severity of illness may impact upon the patient's capacity to benefit, it will not, alone, determine capacity to benefit. A severely ill patient with no capacity to benefit has no "need" under this definition. *Health care needs* thus reflect the potential ability to benefit from particular interventions, whether curative or preventative. Health care needs represent the distribution in the population of indications for treatment, and must therefore accommodate the range of wider concerns that influence the decision to treat.[9] These include the level of morbidity, the presence of comorbidity, other influences upon the potential to benefit from an intervention, as well as the acceptability of the intervention to the recipient. This can be described at the intimate level of the individual's preferences in relation to her/his own perception of her/his problem.

With either of these definitions, the principle often advocated is one of equal access for those in equal need, with the implication being that those with greater need have greater access and those with less need have less access. The concern has generally been with access rather than health itself or the use of health services. Although either of these latter could provide alternative criteria, they would mean that individual preferences about whether or not they wish to receive treatment would not be relevant. Hence this section concentrates upon equal access for equal need. Even within a priority-setting basis of equal access for equal need, however, the precise equity criterion will differ depending upon the way in which funds are allocated between those with greater and lesser needs. The basis of equal access for equal need could either involve meeting all the greatest needs and none of the lesser ones, or it could involve some provision for all needs, but lesser provision for lesser needs (the latter seeming to fit in with Mooney's suggestions[10]). In any case it encompasses the concepts of both vertical and horizontal equity, where horizontal equity entails the equal treatment of those equal in some characteristic – need in this case – and vertical equity entails treating differently those, in this case, with different needs.

Informing the Extent of Priority Setting

Effectiveness is central to the determination of *health care needs*, and thus to priority setting on this basis. It is clearly not necessary to consider the priority for ineffective interventions, which anyway should have no important advocates. Although this is obvious, studies of medical practice consistently find disturbing variations in rates of treatment and in the appropriateness of much hospital care.[11] These variations make it difficult to determine the extent to which the rationing of effective care may be required.

Clinicians' judgements concerning the benefits of treating or not treating are based upon the presence of particular indications. One explanation for the wide variations that exist in clinical practice is that these judgements differ from clinician to clinician. Detailed work conducted in the USA primarily by researchers at the RAND Corporation suggests that, in certain clinical areas, the proportion of inappropriate interventions may be high.[12] The potential for substitution between ineffective and effective interventions is therefore high. Indeed the full potential for such substitution could indicate that rationing by effectiveness would be equivalent to very little rationing at all.

It may also be, however, that more care is effective than can be afforded with the resources available for health services. This is particularly the case where care which appears to be effective, say on the basis of clinical judgement, is a contender for resources even in the absence of good "scientific" evidence to this end. In practice, this may be the case with much of the health care currently provided.

The scale of rationing required to meet current needs is not known. There is not good information about either the proportion of the care currently delivered that is effective, or the proportion of people not currently receiving care who would benefit from treatment. In time, modern epidemiology, in harness with health services research, may provide evidence about both of these vital statistics.

SETTING EXPLICIT PRIORITIES ON THE BASIS OF NEED

Need has formed a basis for unacknowledged rationing within the NHS since its inception.[13] Both the use of the GP as gatekeeper to secondary care and the rationing of care by the use of waiting lists are based on allocating resources on the basis of need (however defined). For example, waiting lists embody the notion that those patients who will not die if they are not treated immediately (elective surgery patients, primarily) can be asked to wait for treatment until there are the resources to provide that treatment. Further, within this group of patients, some (those less severely ill or disabled) have in the past been asked to wait longer than others (those with greater disability or illness). Treatment has been largely allocated on the basis of the relative need between different patients. In recent years there have been attempts to make more explicit the values that are incorporated into the level of urgency assigned to particular patients on waiting lists. For example, there have been attempts in Salisbury to allocate positions on the waiting list using a formula based on the progress of the disease, pain, disability or dependence on others, loss of usual occupation and time spent waiting.[14] Despite such attempts, the use of waiting lists as a means of rationing by need has become, increasingly, politically unacceptable in the UK.[9,15]

Need as a basis for explicit priority setting can be considered in two ways: globally through population-based proxies purporting to summarise the composite of individual morbidity; or specifically through the epidemiological examination of the distribution of particular diseases. While global epidemiology has traditionally assessed inequity in health, with studies continuing to document differences in sickness by social class,[2,3] the major use of global epidemiology in terms of priority setting has been via the measures developed for the broad allocation of health care resources. In particular, such measures have been used to allocate resources for hospital and community health services to regional health authorities in England, and within the regions of England, and the countries of Scotland, Wales, and Northern Ireland (Resource Allocation Working Party formula (RAWP)[16]).

Since the RAWP Report was published in 1976,[16] there has been considerable debate about the kind of equity that is being sought in such formulae.[17–19] RAWP interpreted its terms of reference to mean equalising "opportunity of access for people at equal risk", and in practice resource allocation formulae aim to equalise resources for defined populations taking account of differences in the risk of their requiring health services. Much has been written about the RAWP formula,[20–22] but it is unlikely that it can form a way forward in the priority-setting debate as it is based upon a definition of need – *health needs* (burden of disease) as opposed to *health care needs* (capacity to benefit) – which is increasingly accepted as inadequate for the purposes of priority setting.

The remainder of this section therefore focuses on the potential for setting specific priorities through the epidemiological examination of the distribution of particular diseases. Disease epidemiology can offer a combination of information concerning disease, health service use and effectiveness, and is seen as central to health needs assessment by purchasers. The approach is referred to here, and elsewhere, as that of total needs assessment, and it is clear that this approach has been given a pivotal role in the development of purchasing in the NHS market of the UK.

Total Needs Assessment

Working for patients not only introduced an internal market in the UK, but, by separating purchasers from providers, created a group, purchasers, who are expressly responsible for meeting the needs of their populations: *Working for patients* aimed to put "the needs of patients first".[23] Following the implementation of *Working for patients*, there was a flurry of conferences and published papers, particularly in public health medicine, heralding the centrality of needs assessment in the new market place. Yet it was also clear that there was an impressive dearth of pertinent evidence with which to inform these assessments of need. In particular this problem arose because, although there was information about the general health status of the population, there was remarkably little evidence about the need among populations for particular forms of health care. Previous research activity had been concerned almost exclusively with the need for health rather than the distribution of those who could be expected to benefit from an intervention.[9,24]

Since the early 1990s, needs have been assessed for many conditions. Not only have there been specific assessments of need for particular treatments (for example, see Stevens and Raftery[25,26]), however, but the notion of assessing need has also been applied to the formation of clinical guidelines, and to the formation of national health care targets. Clinical guidelines have tended to relate to the availability of effective treatment for particular conditions. For example, guidelines for dialysis have been developed so that provision is recommended for those patients with greater potential for benefit.[27] The targets contained in *The health of the nation*[28] were also based primarily on need, with the specific use of three criteria. First, that the area of health to be targeted should be one that results in a large burden of illness; second, that effective intervention should be available; and third, that there should be the possibility of quantifying targets for the area of health.[10]

There has, however, been relatively little thought about how the collection of large quantities of information about need could be used in priority setting across different conditions or treatments. In tandem there seems to have been a lack of willingness to engage in discussions about making choices. If, however, information on need is to provide a means of setting priorities, there must be some basis upon which to decide between different forms of need – in practice, different forms of "effective" care. As Mooney states, on this point the literature is exceedingly quiet.[10]

Mooney suggests three options for using information on need (defined as capacity to benefit) as a basis for priority setting.[10] First, he suggests the possibility of allocating resources, pro rata, with needs. Second, he suggests the possibility of using needs assessments merely to provide an ordinal ranking of the resources to be allocated to each area – that is, conditions with the greatest needs should get more resources than conditions with lesser needs. In this case, however, as Mooney states, there is no basis for deciding how much should be spent on each need. Third, he suggests the option of using cardinal weights to reflect the relative importance of the needs of different conditions.[10] Presumably, in order to maintain equity once this allocation had been carried out, there would be some form of random allocation within each "need category".

A further option would be to meet all of the greatest individual needs before attempting to meet the lesser individual needs, for example providing all treatments which bestow 30 additional years of life before meeting those where only 6 months of life are gained. Such a process would entail comparing the available budget with the costs of treating all patients at the different levels of need.

A Critique of Total Needs Assessment

Disease-based Needs Assessment as Technical Priority Setting

Early enthusiasm for needs assessment by purchasers in the UK has waned because of the enormity of the task, the time required, and its irrelevance to purchasers' immediate pressures and the way in which purchaser performance is assessed. (Two criteria loom larger than any others for purchasers in the UK. These are to reduce waiting times and to improve performance on the "efficiency index", which requires purchasers to contract each year to reduce the unit cost of each Finished Consultant Episode. Neither is influenced by needs assessment.) Further, there has been extensive criticism of the needs assessment approach to priority setting by some UK economists.[10,29,30] Mooney, for example, observes:

> One of the potentially great advantages for needs assessors is that while they are engaged in such exercises, they do not have to face up to the difficult and demanding choices involved in priority setting of services. Caught up in the apparently laudable task of assessing needs, the key choice that is required is what data to collect. (Mooney,[10] p.39)

There are formidable difficulties in trying to set priorities from assessment of needs, for example:[10]

- What type of effectiveness is at issue? Is it clinical effectiveness (for example, the lowering of blood pressure), or is it effectiveness in terms of the perceptions of the patient?
- Is it just health benefits that are of interest, or should other benefits such as information provision be included?
- What weights (if any) ought to be attached to social factors such as the ability to return to work, or the ability to drive, or the ability to care for dependants?

Each of these theoretical value judgements will impact upon the type of equity that is achieved through health needs assessment. Beyond these value judgements, though, are methodological and practical details in the formation of health measures which will also affect the extent to which equity is obtained. These problems are discussed in Chapter 5 in relation to the use of QALYs and apply equally to the use of a common outcome measure for assessing "need".

Like most forms of technical priority setting, conducting needs assessment carries the implication of large requirements for data. Oregon's second list (see Chapter 2) essentially based priorities for a large number of condition/treatment pairs upon need (defined as capacity to benefit).[31] Just as with the initial list, which had its basis in cost–utility analysis, the second list was heavily criticised for the quality of the data incorporated.[32-34] The alternative to a broad assessment of many condition/treatment pairs, as in Oregon, would be to combine individually conducted needs assessments in a piecemeal manner, perhaps in the manner of QALY league tables (see Chapter 5). Unfortunately this is likely to lead to similar problems to those associated with QALY league tables;[35,36] for example, assessments of need may be conducted at different times, in different locations, and using non-comparable measures of need (including effectiveness) which may incorporate different values. Each of these factors may make comparison difficult across different assessments of need.

Disease-based Needs Assessment: Equity and Efficiency

Needs assessment involves setting priorities on the basis of health needs (severity of illness) and/or health care needs (capacity to benefit). It is, however, generally conducted without regard to relative cost. As Stevens and Gabbay summarise:

> In the context of the National Health Service Review, 'need' may best be defined as the ability to benefit from 'health care', which depends both on morbidity and on the effectiveness of care. (Stevens and Gabbay,[7] p.20)

Although there are some exceptions, in which information about cost-effectiveness has been included in published needs assessments,[25,26] the approach of assessing need has in general provided a natural target for economists because the resultant priorities are not influenced by cost and hence are not concerned with efficiency:[10]

> If we do not allow for costs in priority setting, then this would mean that if some new technology allowed heart transplants to be carried out at one tenth of their current cost, then such a change would have no effect on priorities in health care. (Mooney,[10] p.38)

Indeed, much of the criticism by economists of the needs assessment approach arises from the fact that the approach does not focus on maximising the available benefit. There is a normative question, however, as to whether the focus should be on efficiency – which combines effectiveness information with cost – or on equity in terms of need – which (for need defined as capacity to benefit, at least) is concerned with information on effectiveness only. Both approaches were tried in Oregon (see Chapter 2), but the first list, based on efficiency, was rejected. This list produced what seemed to be absurd results, whereby conditions of low need (but low cost) were ranked above conditions of high need (but high cost). The revised list ignored cost and was instead based on the principle of meeting all the greatest individual needs before attempting to meet the lesser individual needs. Cost was allowed to influence the results only in the final re-ranking by commissioners of "out-of-place" items on the list.[31] This second list was generally considered much more acceptable and was retained.

To criticise needs assessment on the basis that it does not meet efficiency objectives is, in a sense, to set up a straw man. Needs assessment is concerned with equity rather than efficiency, and hence cannot be expected to lead to an efficient outcome. Whether the precise equity objectives that needs assessment aims to meet are the desired ones is a different issue. While some may favour treating those with greatest capacity to benefit before treating those with lesser capacity to benefit, others may hold different equity objectives which may or may not conflict with these.

CONCLUSION: NEED

Total needs assessment could, potentially, provide a means of setting priorities based on the relative need for different treatments. In this context, need must inevitably be seen as a relative concept. (The extent of absolute need for health in any society may, of course, go far beyond the level at which such needs could be met.) To date, however, the issue of setting priorities between different needs has not generally been addressed. Rather, the expectations created by assessing total needs, that such needs both could and should be met, have generally remained. If needs assessment is to provide a useful basis for explicit priority setting, these issues must be examined in greater depth.

The advantage of needs assessment for priority setting is that it must, by definition, take a population perspective. Hence a population view of the health care needs for cataract surgery, for example, would allow one to consider those levels of indications that would approximate to certain levels of relief for the entire population at risk. Rationing would then be applied not at the margins, in denying the last case in the lottery of varying indications for particular treatments, but to the entire population. Such a population perspective is based on the equity principle of equal access to interventions for those in similar predicaments. This notion is discussed further in Chapter 9, in which the model of health care requirements, which provides an attempt to combine needs-based equity objectives with efficiency objectives, is also discussed.

EQUITY AND AGE-BASED RATIONING

The debate over rationing by age has been conducted mainly in the USA, with little discussion in the UK of rationing explicitly by age. Policies advocating age-based rationing may have a number of different ethical bases. These will be discussed below, focusing in particular on the writings of two individuals: Daniel Callahan and Norman Daniel. The arguments of these two authors are summarised below, but it is recommended that the original texts are read by those who wish to appreciate the subtlety of the complex arguments that have been developed.

THE PHILOSOPHICAL BASIS FOR AGE-BASED RATIONING

Ethicists' discussions of rationing by age have slightly different bases for their arguments, but the philosophical underpinnings are similar. Crudely, the justification for age-based rationing (discussed below) is that each individual would theoretically have a greater benefit over their lifetime if the resources currently used to extend life when they are elderly were instead used earlier in life.[37] Moral justifications for age-based rationing are thus directly concerned with the use of age as a means of choosing who should receive care. It is noticeable that the justifications for rationing by age are *not* related to the use of age as a proxy for the assessment of outcome or need, although much of the opposition to age-based rationing assumes that this is the case.

Two names are particularly connected with the debate about age-based rationing in the USA. Daniel Callahan and Norman Daniel have both written extensively on this subject. The views of each are discussed below, although it is not possible to do full justice to the detailed arguments presented by these authors.

Callahan argues for treating the elderly as a different and special group as regards rationing.[38] The fastest growing age group in the USA is that of those aged over 85, with numbers rising at the rate of about 10% every two years.[39] Callahan also provides estimates of the proportion of the elderly in the population by the year 2040 (21%) and the proportion of health care expenditure they are likely to consume (45%).[39] At the same time as the elderly population is growing, the proportion of younger working people is expected to decline.[38] Callahan links these figures with the expected high costs of life-extending treatment in the last year of life and the increasing amount that can be done for this age group and concludes that society will simply not be able to provide this amount of health care.[38,39]

Callahan combines his arguments over the need to ration care for the elderly with the contention that current programmes that focus on life-extending care are inadequate in providing for the real needs of this group, which are to do with care rather than cure.[39] Callahan's own view is that "the future goal of medicine in the care of the aged should be that of improving the quality of life, not in seeking ways to extend that life" (Callahan,[39] p.127). On a practical level he is concerned with the lack of decent provision of long-term care, while, in more abstract terms, he wants a rethink among US society of the meaning of ageing and death. He supports the view that it is possible to have a meaningful old age that is limited in time, and advocates a culture that provides a more supportive context for ageing and death.[39]

Callahan's practical proposals call for a better balance between caring and curing in the elderly population,[38] with the primary aim of health care being to avoid premature death. Once the natural lifespan has been reached the relief of suffering should be all important.[39]

Callahan's own view is that this natural lifespan is likely to end in the late 70s or early 80s, at which time the individual should have had time, typically, to accomplish the opportunities they have been afforded in life.[39] It is interesting that Callahan also supports the notion of rationing by age because it provides a universal standard, and is comprehensible on the basis of common sense.[39]

It has been said by some commentators that Daniel's Prudential Lifespan Account rests on a stronger philosophical and moral basis than Callahan's proposal.[40] Daniel[41,42] shows that, under restrictive conditions, age as a basis for rationing is morally permissible. He argues that health care is of moral importance because it helps to ensure that individuals have the chance to enjoy the normal opportunities in their society. He refers to this as fair equality of opportunity.[42] Daniel also states that, within lives, different tasks are central at different times, for example pursuit of a career and family in adult years, and that "prudent deliberation . . . would attempt to assure individuals a fair chance at enjoyment of the normal opportunity range for each life-stage" (Daniel,[42] p.104). Consequently, he believes that the rationing of health care should respect the importance of the opportunity range at each stage of life. He uses an appropriate veil of ignorance from behind which the prudent decision can be made, and concludes, although not with complete confidence, that giving greater emphasis to increasing the chance of having a normal lifespan would be more prudent than giving greater emphasis to extending the normal lifespan.[42]

Daniel illustrates his points by comparing age-based rationing with a lottery scheme.[41] He assumes that everyone will catch some illness at age 50. There are only the resources fully to cure half the people, with a cure meaning that people live until age 100. One option is to have a lottery to make this decision. The other is to give everyone half a cure, so that they live until age 75. While the latter option might seem intuitively fairer, or more equitable, this is not the basis that Daniel uses to support his argument. Instead, as stated, he uses the notion of a prudent individual who would, as Daniel illustrates using different rules, be more likely to choose the option of living until 75 than choosing the option of dying immediately or living until 100. Thus the prudent individual, where resources are scarce, would choose age-based rationing over rationing by lottery.

Daniel extends his argument from the individual, who would prefer to use resources earlier than later, to age cohorts. He does this by viewing health insurance as a savings scheme whereby resources are deferred from one point in life to another, and as a cohort, decisions can be made about the relative weight given to care at different ages. Daniel is clear that his approach does not provide a general sanction for rationing by age. First, resources must be limited, and second, rationing by age can only be applicable where it is part of the design of a basic institution which distributes resources over the lifetime of individuals. Thus his argument does not justify the piecemeal use of criteria based on age.[42]

AGE-BASED RATIONING: A CRITIQUE

Implicit and Explicit Rationing by Age

There is a misapprehension, common in North America, that age discrimination in the NHS is "both universally practised and in some degree officially sanctioned" (Grimley Evans,[43] p.118). Although there is some evidence that age has been used, in a relatively ad hoc manner, as an implicit criterion for allocating care, age as an explicit basis for priority setting has not been taken particularly seriously. In fact the British Medical Association (BMA), while accepting the need to ration, stated explicitly in 1992 that patients should not be denied medical diagnosis and treatment on the basis of advanced age.[44]

Despite this official position, however, it has been asserted that age has formed the basis of implicit rationing of care in the UK in the past.[45] Discussion of age-based rationing in the UK has particularly focused on the implicit rationing to the elderly of dialysis for those with end-stage renal disease. For example, Wing quotes figures that in 1982 only 8% of new dialysis patients in the UK were aged over 65,[46] with this figure being much lower than those of other European countries.[46] One study has shown that age-based rationing is not justified on the anticipation of a poor prognosis for these patients.[47] Age-related policies have also been found in coronary care units across the UK. Of 134 units replying to a survey, 26 stated that they operated age-related policies. Of these, two had an upper limit of age

65, seven an upper limit of age 70, 14 an upper limit of age 75 and two an upper limit of age 80.[48] Although the survey did not ask why these policies were administered, some respondents added comments stating their reasons. These included lack of beds, the frailty of older patients and the belief that younger patients derive more benefit from care.

It is not only in the UK, however, that age appears to have been used as an implicit rationing criterion. There have also been examples quoted from the USA of apparent rationing on the basis of age.[49,50] One study researching into the care of breast cancer patients of different ages found, using logistic regression, that both age and comorbidity status independently and significantly affected the treatment received by patients.[49] For example, stage I and II patients with no, or mild, comorbidity were compared across different age groups. Among those aged between 50 and 69 appropriate surgery was received by 96%, but for those aged over 70 appropriate surgery was received by only 83%. The authors concluded that management of patients was conducted on the basis of chronological age as well as prognosis.[49]

Age as Technical Priority Setting?

Limiting treatments on the basis of age appears to be a form of technical priority setting in that it applies limits on the basis of rules suggested by philosophical reasoning. Particularly if the philosophical reasoning can suggest a specific limit, such as Callahan's "natural lifespan" of the late 70s or early 80s, the means of priority setting seems to be very technical. Levinsky in fact makes the point that a categorical criterion such as age might be appealing because it is clear and easy to administer, although in his view this ease of application is a disadvantage.[37]

Some of the criticisms that have been made of rationing care between individuals on the basis of quality-adjusted life-years, might equally be applied to a criterion of rationing by age. In particular, given the heterogeneous nature of individuals, the "natural lifespan" may differ considerably between individuals – in other words, some individuals may reach the end of their "natural lifespan" at a time considerably earlier than their late 70s, while others may not reach such a time until well past their early 80s. This may be both in terms of accomplishing the available opportunities and in terms of the individual's health. There is another difficulty: the opportunities available to individuals may differ significantly, with further potential implications for rationing by age.

There has also been disagreement with Callahan's arguments that the majority of individuals in the USA incur high costs in the final years of their lives.[40] This has raised questions about whether reducing curative treatments from the end of the "natural lifespan" would have any effects on the amount of health care purchased, with some commentators stating that it would do little to slow the costs of health care.[40] If rationing were to be required beyond this "natural lifespan" there is the issue of by how much to reduce this figure.[40]

In practice, elements of pluralistic bargaining might well be built into such a scheme in terms of making decisions about the age at which limits might be set and whether this should be the same age for all interventions. There is also a question as to whether age-based rationing is generally considered to be acceptable. On the basis of 719 interviews conducted in Cardiff that looked at a number of different personal characteristics as bases for limiting care, a survey found the clearest consensus to be that younger people should have preference over older people.[51] This work did not, however, consider explicitly the acceptability of rationing on the basis of personal characteristics compared with the acceptability of rationing on the basis of treatment characteristics.

Age-based Rationing: Equity and Efficiency

There is much discussion over the justice, or otherwise, of age-based rationing. While the general principle appears to be one of equality of access to health care over a lifetime, the philosophical basis also incorporates the notion that cohorts of individuals would have a greater benefit over their lifetime if resources that could be used to extend life when they are elderly were instead used earlier in life.[37]

Much of the discussion of the equity basis of limiting care on the basis of age comes from the seeming assumption that one group of individuals – the elderly – is worth less than another – the young. A particular danger appears to be that, by singling out one group for special treatment, the door is opened for treating other groups differently, for example those of different sex or race.[52] Daniel, however, contrasts rationing by age with rationing on the basis of, say, race or sex, and concludes that there are differences, because rationing by race or sex crosses personal boundaries, whereas rationing by age only looks as if personal boundaries are crossed if a "time-slice perspective" is taken (Daniel,[42] p.97). Old age is something that affects all individuals, unlike, say, race or sex. Limiting resources on the basis of age, Daniel maintains, would not lead to inequality if the scheme is systematically applied across the whole lifespan.[41] One interesting problem with this reasoning, pointed out by Jecker, is that age-based rationing would disproportionately affect women (who generally live longer lives than men). She therefore concludes that age-based rationing would be inequitable.[53] In making this assertion Jecker assumes that a similar age criterion would be set across both sexes, and by implication across all sectors of society. It is interesting to question whether it would be more inequitable to have different criteria for the different sexes – and maybe for other characteristics as well – or whether it is more inequitable to have the same criterion for all.

Further criticism of the equity basis of rationing by age has come from those who believe that support for the use of age is based on expectations that it will correlate with outcome.[43,54] For example, Grimley Evans states that he objects to the use of age in this way, commenting that if social class were used on the same basis the result would be outrage.[43] He also states that age will contribute little to the prediction of outcome and that thus its use is unscientific.[55]

The intention of Daniel and Callahan is not to justify rationing by age on the basis of perceived poorer outcome among the elderly. For them this is not the relevant issue. Because, however, the use of an age criterion would almost certainly conflict at times with expectations of outcome, it would probably be difficult to operate in practice. Where a clinician considers that it is possible to provide an elderly person with a life-extending intervention that is both effective and cost-effective, they are likely to be most unwilling to refuse such treatment purely on the grounds of age. Hence, Siegler is concerned with limiting care to the elderly because it threatens to undermine traditions of clinical medicine, based upon medical need and patient preferences,[56] and Cassel argues that decisions should be made on the basis of prognosis rather than on the basis of age.[57]

Other concerns have also been expressed. The first is mainly applicable to the USA, and is a result of the system of health care there. Age rationing there would not result in extra resources for health care for others in the same way as it would in the UK, as there is no global health budget. Thus reducing the resources available to one group would not mean that those resources were necessarily available to provide health care to other groups. Hence age-based rationing would be unjust.[58] In a sense this is acknowledged by Callahan, who uses the NHS, in part, as an example of what he is advocating.[59] The second concern is that there will be some patients who are able to play the system so that it works in their favour. Thus although the intent might be equitable, the outcome of an age-based rationing scheme would be unfair.[37] Although almost certainly justified, this concern could, however, be applied to any form of rationing, whether implicit or explicit.

It might appear that, in some ways, rationing by age as advocated by Daniel is based on utilitarianism, and thus efficiency, because it is based upon the maximisation of benefit available throughout life. Daniel, however, explicitly states that the basis is not utilitarianism (or efficiency) because that would involve maximising benefit across individuals, whereas his justification is based only upon maximising within individuals.[41] Rationing by age, per se, is unlikely to accord with efficiency objectives (which involve maximising benefit across individuals), except in so far as the cost-effectiveness of providing different treatments varies with age.

CONCLUSION: AGE-BASED RATIONING

The arguments for age-based rationing have a detailed philosophical basis and are well thought out. This is in contrast to many of the arguments for basing priorities on need (see above). Despite this, however, explicit rationing by age appears to be much less acceptable than priority setting on the basis of need. Certainly, there is opposition to the notion from the BMA, and the debate on age-based rationing, which has been relatively extensive in the USA, has made little impact on the UK. It seems that, in the UK, it is more acceptable to think about priorities in terms of the treatments that should be a priority than about the people that should be a priority. Whereas age-based rationing requires the identification and isolation of a particular group who would be deprived of "curing" treatment (but not of "caring" treatment), rationing by need allows for the possibility of treatment for all types of individual, depending only upon the particular need that they exhibit.

CONCLUSIONS

This chapter has reviewed two distinctive and controversial examples of particular equity objectives in terms of their potential impact on priority setting. Beyond these two contrasting bases are undoubtedly many other options that could equally claim to be a just basis for rationing. These would include rationing on perhaps the most equitable basis of all: random allocation through a lottery.[60-62]

Priority setting in the UK, however, is currently most likely to be influenced by the principle of equity according to need, with need (and/or effectiveness) both advocated in official policy documents,[23] and forming the historical basis of the NHS. This is also the principle which appears to have gained greatest acceptance elsewhere. In both Oregon and New Zealand, despite the very different approaches to priority setting, support has been given to providing treatments for which the patient has capacity to benefit, thus meeting "need" as defined in this manner. In Oregon treatments were ranked on the basis of capacity to benefit, with those treatments that appeared to provide greatest capacity to benefit being ranked most highly.[31] In New Zealand, the framework upon which priority setting is based contains, as its first criterion, that the treatments which are resourced should provide benefit.[63] The principle, however, suffers from the same issues of practicality as the methods of economic evaluation discussed in Chapter 5: there is a constant need for large quantities of data which must be updated whenever there are changes to medical technology.

In contrast, the notion of rationing explicitly by age has largely remained a theoretical option. This is despite the apparent existence of implicit rationing upon this basis, and despite the fact that age-based rationing would undoubtedly be considerably cheaper than other forms of technical rationing, requiring much fewer data. Although the moral arguments for age-based rationing have been thoroughly developed, many question its justice on the basis that it does not take into account the need for treatment. Setting priorities on the basis of personal characteristics, rather than on the basis of the characteristics of the treatment, is also offensive to many. Hence, age-based rationing may be less useful as a way forward than other equity bases for setting priorities.

It is clear even from this detailed examination of two options, that different equity bases for setting priorities will almost certainly conflict with one another. Perhaps, therefore, the major means of reducing confusion would be to conduct further research into what individuals mean by equity and on what sort of equity basis they would prefer priority setting to be based.

REFERENCES

1. Mooney G. Equity in health care: confronting the confusion. *Effective Health Care* 1983; **1**: 179–84.
2. Black D, Morris JN, Smith C, Townsend P. The Black report. In: *Inequalities in health*. Penguin Books, London, 1992: 31–218.
3. Whitehead M. The health divide. In: *Inequalities in health*. Penguin Books, London, 1992: 219–437.
4. Matthew GK. Measuring need and evaluating services. In: McLachlan G, ed. *Portfolio for health. The role and programme of the DHSS in health services research*. Oxford University Press, London, 1971.
5. Hunter DJW, McKee M. Patients' interests or resource allocation. *BMJ* 1993; **306**: 656–7.
6. Stevens A, Raftery J. Introduction. In: Stevens A, Raftery J, eds. *Health care needs assessment. The epidemiologically based needs assessment reviews*. Radcliffe Medical Press, Oxford, 1994: 11–30.
7. Stevens A, Gabbay J. Needs assessment needs assessment. *Health Trends* 1991; **23**(1): 20–3.
8. Bradshaw JS. A taxonomy of social need. In: McLachlan G, ed. *Problems and progress in medical care: essays on current research*. 7th series edition.

Oxford University Press, Oxford, 1972.

9. Frankel SJ. Health needs, health-care requirements, and the myth of infinite demand. *Lancet* 1991; **337**: 1588–90.

10. Mooney G. *Key issues in health economics*. Harvester Wheatsheaf, New York, 1994.

11. Andersen TG, Mooney G. *The challenges of medical practice variations*. Macmillan, Basingstoke, 1990.

12. Leape LL, Edward-Park R, Solomon D, Chassin MR, Kosecoff J, Brook RH. Does inappropriate use explain small-area variations in the use of health care services? *J Am Med Assoc* 1990; **263**(5): 669–72.

13. Frankel S, West R. *Rationing and rationality in the National Health Service. The persistence of waiting lists*. Macmillan, Basingstoke, 1993.

14. Tudor Edwards R. An economic perspective of the Salisbury waiting list points scheme. In: Malek M, ed. *Setting priorities in health care*. John Wiley, Chichester, 1994: 59–689.

15. Coast J. The role of economic evaluation in setting priorities for elective surgery. *Health Policy* 1993; **24**: 243–57.

16. Department of Health and Social Security. *Sharing resources for health in England. Report of the Resource Allocation Working Party (The RAWP report)*. HMSO, London, 1976.

17. Buxton MJ, Klein RE. *Allocating health resources: a commentary on the Report of the Resource Allocation Working Party (Royal Commission on the National Health Service, Research Paper 2)*. HMSO, London, 1978.

18. Mooney GH. *Economics, medicine and health care*. Harvester Wheatsheaf, London, 1986.

19. Bebbington AC, Davies B. Territorial need indicators: a new approach. *J Soc Pol* 1980; **9**: 145–68.

20. Sheldon TA, Davey Smith G, Bevan G. Weighting in the dark: resource allocation in the new NHS. *BMJ* 1993; **306**: 835–9.

21. Bevan G. Ways of seeing: explaining variation in use of acute hospital services. *Int J Epidemiol* 1995; **24**: S103–8.

22. Carr-Hill R, Sheldon T. Rationality and the use of formulae in the allocation of resources to health care. *J Public Health Med* 1992; **14**(2): 117–26.

23. Department of Health. *Working for patients*. HMSO, London, 1989.

24. Frankel SJ. The epidemiology of indications. *J Epidemiol Community Health* 1991; **45**(4): 257–9.

25. Stevens A, Raftery J, eds. *Health care needs assessment. The epidemiologically based needs assessment reviews. Volume 1*. Radcliffe Medical Press, Oxford, 1994.

26. Stevens A, Raftery J, eds. *Health care needs assessment. The epidemiologically based needs assessment reviews. Volume 2*. Radcliffe

Medical Press, Oxford, 1994.

27. Moss AH, Rettig RA, Cassel CK. A proposal for guidelines for patient acceptance to and withdrawal from dialysis: a follow-up to the IOM report. *ANNA J* 1993; **20**(5): 557–61.

28. Department of Health. *The health of the nation. A strategy for health in England*. HMSO, London, 1992.

29. Donaldson C. Economics, public health and health care purchasing: reinventing the wheel. *Health Policy* 1995; **33**(2): 79–90.

30. Mooney G, Gerard K, Donaldson C, Farrar S. *Priority setting in purchasing. Some practical guidelines*. NAHAT, Birmingham, 1992.

31. Oregon Health Services Commission. *Prioritization of Health Services. A report to the Governor and Legislature*. Oregon Health Services Commission, 1991.

32. Nelson RM, Drought T. Justice and the moral acceptability of rationing medical care: the Oregon experiment. *J Med Philos* 1992; **17**: 97–117.

33. Maynard A. On the Oregon trail. *Health Service J* 1991; **23 May**: 28.

34. Honigsbaum F. *Who shall live? Who shall die? – Oregon's health financing proposals*. King's Fund College, London, 1991.

35. Gerard K, Mooney G. *QALY League Tables: three points for concern – goal difference counts*. Health Economics Research Unit, Aberdeen, 1992.

36. Mason J, Drummond M, Torrance G. Some guidelines on the use of cost effectiveness league tables. *BMJ* 1993; **306**: 570–2.

37. Levinsky NG. Age as a criterion for rationing health care. *N Engl J Med* 1990; **322**(25): 1813–15.

38. Callahan D. Should health care for the elderly be rationed? *Coronary Artery Dis* 1993; **4**: 393–4.

39. Callahan D. Aging and the ends of medicine. *Ann N Y Acad Sci* 1988; **530**: 125–32.

40. Hoopes R. When it's time to leave. Can society set an age limit for health care? *Modern Maturity* 1988; **August–September**: 38–43.

41. Daniel N. Rationing by age. In: *Am I my parents' keeper? An essay on justice between the young and the old*. Oxford University Press, New York, 1988: 83–102.

42. Daniel N. Am I my parents' keeper? In: *Just health care*. Cambridge University Press, Cambridge, 1985: 86–113.

43. Grimley Evans J. Age and equality. *Ann N Y Acad Sci* 1988; **530**: 118–24.

44. British Medical Association. Rationing and allocation of health care resources. In: *Medical ethics today*. BMJ, London, 1993: 299–316.

45. Baker R. The inevitability of health care rationing: a case study of rationing in the British National Health Service. In: Strosberg MA, Weiner JM, Baker R, Fein IA, eds. *Rationing America's medical care: the Oregon plan and beyond*. The Brookings Institution, Washington, DC,

1992: 208–29.

46. Wing AJ. Why don't the British treat more patients with kidney failure? *BMJ* 1983; **287**: 1157–8.

47. Taube DH, Winder EA, Ogg CS et al. Successful treatment of middle aged and elderly patients with end stage renal disease. *BMJ* 1983; **286**: 2018–20.

48. Dudley NJ, Burns E. The influence of age on policies for admission and thrombolysis in coronary care units in the United Kingdom. *Age Ageing* 1992; **21**: 95–8.

49. Greenfield S, Blanco DM, Elashoff RM, Ganz PA. Patterns of care related to age of breast cancer patients. *J Am Med Assoc* 1987; **257**: 2766–70.

50. Samet J, Hunt WC, Key C, Humble CG, Goodwin JS. Choice of cancer therapy varies with age of patient. *J Am Med Assoc* 1986; **255**: 3385–90.

51. Vetter N, Lewis P, Farrow S, Charny M. Who would you choose to save? *Health Service J* 1989; **99**: 976–7.

52. Childress JF. Ensuring care, respect and fairness for the elderly. *Hastings Center Rep* 1984; **October**: 27–31.

53. Jecker NS. Age-based rationing and women. *J Am Med Assoc* 1991; **266**(21): 3012–15.

54. Kilner JF. Age criteria in medicine. Are the medical justifications ethical? *Arch Intern Med* 1989; **149**: 2343–6.

55. Grimley Evans J. Aging and rationing. *BMJ* 1991; **303**: 869–70.

56. Siegler M. Should age be a criterion in health care? *Hastings Center Rep* 1984; **October**: 24–7.

57. Cassel CK. Issues of age and chronic care: another argument for health care reform. *J Am Geriatr Soc* 1992; **40**: 404–9.

58. Battin MP. Age rationing and the just distribution of health care: is there a duty to die? *Ethics* 1987; **97**: 317–40.

59. Callahan D. Setting limits. *Medical goals in an aging society*. Simon and Schuster, New York, 1987.

60. Kilner JF. *Who lives? Who dies? Ethical criteria in patient selection*. Yale University Press, New Haven, 1990.

61. Hope T, Springings D, Crisp R. "Not clinically indicated": patients' interests or resource allocation? *BMJ* 1993; **306**: 379–81.

62. Broome J. Fairness versus doing the most good. *Hastings Center Rep* 1994; **July–August**: 36–9.

63. National Advisory Committee on Core Health and Disability Support Services. *Core Services for 1994/95*. National Advisory Committee on Core Health and Disability Support Services, Wellington, 1993.

PART FOUR

Pluralistic Bargaining and Public Participation

CHAPTER SEVEN

BEN TOTH

Public Participation: An Historical Perspective

This chapter reviews public participation in the organisation of health care from an historical perspective. History is useful not so much for illuminating the past, but as a way of identifying the forces that shape our present position. In considering the development of medical services since the late eighteenth century a number of themes are apparent. First, although the nature of what we recognise as the public and the medical profession varies, the relationship between medicine and the public is important at every period. Secondly, since the late nineteenth century, but particularly in the twentieth, health services have been recognised as socially desirable, and publicly funded health services have been increasingly provided. Yet the public itself has had little part to play in deciding the nature or organisation of these services.

An interpretation of this apparent paradox can be suggested immediately. Table 7.1 displays a number of events regarded as fundamental to the development of state health services in Britain in the past 200 years. These events *also* represent cumulative stages toward the fulfilment of the cultural and economic aspirations of doctors. However, it is not necessary to suggest that doctors acted in unison during the period of medical reform. Many doctors resisted reform. Many of the struggles were between groups of doctors. Nor does this chapter suggest that reform was driven solely by a desire to

Priority Setting: The Health Care Debate.
Edited by J. Coast, J. Donovan and S. Frankel.   © 1996 John Wiley & Sons Ltd.

drive out lay perspectives from medicine. The basis of this chapter is that medical aspirations – to coherent professional status – are intertwined with the growth of state medicine, and that this necessarily involved a re-definition downwards of lay authority in health matters.

Table 7.1 Some significant events in the development of health services in Britain

Year	Event
1815	Apothecaries Act
1848	Public Health Act
1858	Compulsory registration of medical practitioners
1875	Public Health Act
1911	National Health Insurance
1919	Creation of the Ministry of Health
1948	Creation of National Health Service

The decline of lay authority was achieved in part through a critique of lay knowledge about health. In sharpening the distinction between medical and lay knowledge the emerging profession developed two themes. First, it populated the public sphere of the nineteenth and twentieth centuries with medical perspectives.[1,2] Second, it sought to organise public assent concerning the distinction between medical and lay knowledge and practice.

To paint a rough but defensible picture, nineteenth-century medical practice was subject to lay authority within its institutions and popular scepticism without. Twentieth-century medicine has reversed both, creating a zone of application within which medical knowledge is relatively unassailable, and has achieved a large measure of public assent concerning its accomplishments and claims to authority. The reversal in the relationship between the public and its doctors might be regarded as the inevitable consequence of medical progress. The ill-defined but expressive notion of progress is more suitable as a topic for analysis than an explanatory resource and the approach adopted here is closer to those studies that argue that the creation and maintenance of distance in the relation between public and profession represent a tactic towards achieving a modern identity for medicine, and not a consequence of achievement or progress.[3]

Lay perspectives were an integral part of late eighteenth-century medicine.[4] For example, many aspects of the clinical organisation of hospitals, including patient admission, were dominated by non-qualified persons,[5] and it was not until the 1880s that consultants firmly gained control of medical appointments and teaching.[6] In the domestic world, which long remained the main locus for healing practices, the authority of popular remedies and therapeutic systems could easily match that of medical practice.[7,8]

Between this medical anti-arcadia and our own time lie a series of revolutions which together constitute modernisation and the creation of the medical profession:[9] professional and legal reform between the 1815 Apothecaries Act and the Medical Act of 1858; sanitary reform and the public health movement in the mid to late nineteenth century; the emergence of scientific medicine in the late nineteenth century; and the publicly funded health provision movement beginning in the late nineteenth century, culminating in the formation of the NHS. It is amongst these revolutions that the modern relationship between public and medicine developed, defining the legitimate areas of lay and medical knowledge, lay and medical authority over the provision of services.

EXISTING ACCOUNTS OF PUBLIC INVOLVEMENT IN HEALTH CARE

There are relatively few accounts of public involvement in health care policy in the twentieth century. Perhaps this simply reflects a real attenuation in public involvement in health care. But the absence might also be attributed to the masking effects of a way of writing history in which the state increasingly stands in for the public as a source of authority. This is particularly true in the case of the NHS, which is portrayed by writers of all political persuasions as a grandiloquent gesture of unique importance. In recycling a myth that accompanied the birth of the NHS, the extent to which it was necessary to create this moment within public opinion has been effaced from accounts of the creation of health services in the twentieth century.[10] Standard accounts of the development of the NHS make little if any reference to the public.[11-14] The focus of these accounts is in the detail of government/professional drama, portrayed against a distant, relatively unchanging, and consequently irrelevant backcloth of public assent.

In questioning a Weberian concept of the modern state, Jacobs provides a detailed account of the way in which the findings of public opinion polls were used by policymakers in the 1930s and 1940s.[15] He concludes that "empirical research on . . . British health policy . . . suggests that public preferences and understandings have extensive influence on detailed policy making".

His text shows that policymakers mobilised the findings of public opinion polls to discredit opposing positions or to support their own. In this limited sense, the findings of public opinion polls were incorporated into Whitehall policy debate. It is uncontroversial to suggest that public opinion polls were used (often created) by Government agencies. But the technology of public opinion polling need not be in conflict with the Weberian bureaucratic state. In fact public opinion polls can be viewed as a product of declining public involvement in the public sphere. This was the case in British health policy, where the high water mark of public involvement in health policy was the popular but short-lived Ministry of Health Watching Council of 1919, some years before the first public opinion polls.

While there is no comprehensive account of the role of the public in the development of public health services, there are a number of case studies focused on public participation in health policy in the twentieth century. A single volume has been devoted to the topic,[16] and elsewhere relevant material is included in Klein and Howlett's study of complaints against doctors.[17] Detailed case studies of planning and policy making in the NHS during the 1970s reveal the extent to which the public were *not* involved in planning at that time.[18,19] It would therefore be desirable to know more about the NHS and its public: to know, for example, about localised public action; about public representation within the Ministry and later Department of Health; about the influence of pressure groups within Parliament and Whitehall; about the alliances between clinicians and pressure groups; about management of consensus within Area and District Health Authority boards; and about the role of the media and medical charities in framing and translating health issues. Such studies would need a more subtle theoretical structure than that available in the Arnstein model, used to describe the possible ways in which the public can interact with bureaucratic organisations.[20] Marks has observed that each health care issue creates its own public.[21] An observation such as this might form the basis for a series of studies on how audiences are created for health care policies. Such an approach would render problematic any attempt to identify a single public with stable and valid opinions about prioritisation or other health issues, but it might make a useful starting point to explore public involvement in health matters.

Recent studies of the development of eighteenth- and nineteenth-century medicine have emphasised the part played by the public at that time. The proximity of lay and medical perspectives can be ascribed to two features of eighteenth-century medicine according to Roy Porter:[22] the high level of self-medication among all classes of society, and the assertive role of upper-class patients in relation to their physicians. A number of authors have analysed the effect of wider changes on the relationship between doctors and their patients in the eighteenth century.[4,23–25] There has been a greater willingness to explore differing perceptions of medical advance held by doctors and the public in the nineteenth century,[26–28] and to explore the profusion of medical systems available to the public.[29]

The rest of the chapter is divided into two broad sections. The first covers lay/medical relations before the formation of the NHS. The second concerns the ways in which the public have been represented within the NHS.

DOCTORS AND THE PUBLIC BEFORE THE NHS

THE MEDICAL PROFESSION AND THE PUBLIC IN THE NINETEENTH CENTURY

The relationship between doctors and the public can be seen as central to the development of medical services in Great Britain.[25,30] From the late eighteenth century doctors made increasing efforts to secure their public against the temptations of quack medicine, an effort which resulted in a publishing boom of popular medical texts written by doctors.[31] The underlying cause was financial. As the number of regular doctors increased they came more into conflict with their irregular counterparts.[32] Loudon has suggested that the period of reform, between 1794 and 1858, during which medicine reinvented itself as a modern profession, arose in part as a result of the public's failure to condemn sufficiently the activities of druggists, a marginal group who began to replace their former trade of wholesale supply of materia medica to pharmacies with a direct retail supply of drugs to the public in the last decades of the eighteenth century.[33]

Broadly speaking, the picture of medicine entering the nineteenth century portrays two strata of relationship between doctor and patient. There is a patron/client level, which Jewson identified for the eighteenth century, but which was regarded as a model upon which a profession might be based until at least 1820.[34] Here the patient was of a higher social standing than his or her doctor, and had clear expectations of the manner in which medical services would be provided. Alongside this was a second unevenly medicalised segment of the population, in which the services provided by doctors were forced to compete with practices whose authorisation lay outside any medical system.

Neither level was capable of supporting the aspiration of reform. Thomas Wakely, founding editor of the *Lancet*, attacked the medical elite, calling them "cowardly . . . dirty-minded bats" [sic][35] because it did not seem to him to offer the institutional means to effect professional reform. At the other end of the medical spectrum, apothecaries had little civil status: their incomes could hardly be described as secure, and in any case were meagre when compared to members of the Royal College,[6] and undistinguished in relation to other tradesmen.[36]

The possibility of medical advance came with the growth of hospital medicine and by adherence to the precepts of scientific methods.[37-40] The eighteenth-century hospital had been organised around a contractual relationship between rich and poor,[41,42] in which the power of hospital boards to decide matters that were later to be defined as requiring purely clinical judgment was considerable.[43] The dominance of lay authority in hospitals can be seen for example in the manner of dealing with patient complaints. Members of the Weekly Board dealt with complaints.[44] These might have come from patients against doctors, patients against patients, doctors against nurses, doctors against hospital cooks, and so on. There is a sense of levelling at work here in which staff and patients fall under the authority of hospitals' patrons. And whereas today it is seen as a great step forward to have a printed complaints policy, in the eighteenth century the Weekly Board might have toured the hospital soliciting complaints while inspecting the wards.

The nineteenth-century hospital began to reinstate poverty within a medical discourse.* Amongst other things, it created a new ordering of the relationship between patients and their illnesses. Simultaneously, clinical space for patients' narratives, and tolerance of practices labelled as non-scientific, decreased.[23,24,45,46]

Despite the growing confidence of medical thought, medical practice in the nineteenth century was constrained by lay authority. In general practice, mutual associations such as the Friendly Societies dominated the lives of general practitioners. The societies and clubs provided medical services to members on a subscription basis. The solution to the restraints placed on medical practice could not have been predicted even by an astute observer in the mid-nineteenth century. Medicine was to become part of state provision. And in return, state medicine was ultimately to release the medical profession from lay domination.

There was little concept of public health or governmental concern for health in the eighteenth century. But from the publication of *Medical Police* in 1798 the fate of countries became tied to the health of its constituent populations, with a special emphasis placed on the link between poverty and ill health.[47] State Medicine is a generic term for governmental intervention in health-related concerns. In Britain it arose at the confluence of a number of initiatives of the 1830s and 1840s, including the sanitary reform movement, the Factory Commission of 1833, and Poor Law Reform. None of the impulses

---

*Foucault dates the origin in France to the eighteenth century.[119]

that created state medicine arose from within organised medicine. Nor were they dominated by medical figures, although marginal medical practitioners like William Farr quickly recognised the value of sanitary reform.[48] Poor Law Reform stemmed from a Royal Commission established in 1832 and chaired by the Bishop of London.[49,50] Sanitary Reform was a middle-class lay movement, in which women played a significant early role.[51]

Greater space for medical perspectives within sanitary reform was created through the appointment of Medical Officers of Health from 1847 onwards, and through the provisions of the Public Health Acts of 1848 and 1875. But like their clinical colleagues, Medical Officers of Health felt constrained by lay authority and by the Local Government Boards' continuing reliance on non-medical inspectors and "unbounded confidence in glorified common sense in matters of medical and hygienic concern" (Newsholme,[52] p.21).

Sanitary reform proceeded through both local and, from 1848, central initiatives, in the form of the General Board of Health (1848–1858), chaired initially by the non-medically qualified Chadwick, and then by Dr John Simon, who became Medical Officer to the Board in 1855 and campaigned for the Parliamentary President of the General Board of Health to be named the Minister of Health. Under Simon's leadership State Medicine flourished in the 1850s and 1860s.[53] In 1871, however, Simon's department was absorbed into the Local Government Board, and subsequently the restrictions he felt placed upon him by lay administrators led to his resignation in 1876. Not until the creation of the Ministry of Health in 1919 was there space for medicine in the higher echelons of state power.

TOWARDS A STATE MEDICAL SERVICE

By the early twentieth century the need for reformation and reorganisation of hospital services became a focus of a quite widespread concern.[54] Medical Officers of Health argued for the extension of state medical services. But it is doubtful if the successive steps taken towards that goal would have occurred if the wider medical profession had opposed the greater intervention of state organisation in medical arrangements. In this context The National

Health Insurance Act of 1911 (NHI)[55] played an enabling role, for it broke down the conventions embodied in Poor Law medical service[56] and revealed, to the future leaders of the medical profession at least, the benefits of enlightened self-interest. The 1911 Act is often portrayed as crucial to the extension of general practitioner services to working men. But most working men were already covered through Clubs and Friendly Societies.[16,57–59] The main beneficiaries of the Act were evidently General Practitioners. According to Fox:

> medical opposition to the NHI disappeared quickly as, under it, doctors' [i.e. General Practitioners'] incomes rose and their professional autonomy increased because they were freed from what they regarded as the petty restrictions of voluntary group insurance administered by Friendly Societies. (Honigsbaum,[54] p.8)

Within a few years there was a general will to improve the availability of services. Dr Christopher Addison declared that he saw no end to the enlightened co-operation between medicine and the state.[60] The main remaining obstacle, persistent since 1876, was the lack of government machinery led by doctors, to broker the relationship between profession and state.

PUBLIC OPINION AND THE CREATION OF THE MINISTRY OF HEALTH

The campaign for the creation of a Ministry of Health offers the most vivid example of public involvement in the formation of health policy in the twentieth century. But while the extent to which sections of the public became involved in the campaign is impressive by modern standards, the effectiveness of the campaign was ensured by sections of the medical profession and their allies who wished to establish a permanent base for expert medical opinion within government. When Bertrand Dawson wrote "[The Ministry of Health] was brought about by public opinion and not, unfortunately, by medical opinion"[61] he was not praising the public but using the pages of the *British Medical Journal* to rebuke those sections of the profession whose resistance had forced him and others to call upon public support to realise the Ministry.

On the evening of 3 February 1919 Christopher Addison, Bertrand Dawson and Lady Rhondda addressed a demonstration intended to give fresh impetus to the campaign to establish a Ministry of Health. Lady Rhondda welcomed the government's proposal to establish advisory councils:

> The new Ministry would need machinery to keep it in the closest possible touch with public opinion. In this context she thought it most important for the ministry to make use of women (cheers). Beside an advisory council of expert men and women, she would like to see a council composed of ordinary wives and mothers, learning, advising and acting as a link between the ministry and the homes of the country (cheers). Dr Addison, answering questions at the end of the meeting, expressed his willingness to act on Lady Rhondda's suggestion. (*The Times*, 4 February 1919, p.5)

A few days later, on 12 February 1919, Lady Rhondda addressed a meeting at the Royal Institute of Public Health in London. The title of her talk was "Women in the Ministry of Health":

> The promoters of the proposed Ministry must realise that the use to be made of women is, from a health point of view, fundamental. Maternity and infant welfare are of particular importance. This is clearly a service in which women could be of special value, and it is important to know how far women are to be in charge of such a department. (*The Times*, 13 February 1919)

Later that year the legislation creating a Ministry of Health was enacted. The contribution of Lady Rhondda and other prominent leaders of the women's movement to the establishment of the Ministry of Health has not been sufficiently recognised. At a time when many ordinary practitioners opposed the creation of the Ministry senior members of the profession sought to secure the support of the public. Christopher Addison, for example, when he met representatives of the National Union of Women Workers on 16 June 1918 urged them "to continue in their propaganda efforts" (*The Times*, 17 June 1918, p.5)

While the majority of doctors remained cautious about what they regarded as state interference in medicine, Bertrand Dawson saw the creation of a Ministry as a great opportunity for the profession. In lectures (the Cavendish series) and articles (in the *British Medical Journal*) during 1918 Dawson used the titles "the future of the medical profession" and "the Nation's health" interchangeably.[62,63] In these papers he called for a wide expansion of the hospital system, with state support if necessary, to bring the benefits of science to the public, and for a wide measure of unfettered professional control in each area of medicine. "Lay control", he wrote, "is all too strong . . . we believe that a cure for these evils is first and foremost, an enlightened public opinion, made effective through a health ministry, and a series of local health boards. The latter should in no sense control medical men."

In the following year, Margaret Davies wrote to *The Times*:

> The importance of securing the hearty co-operation of the public in the new Ministry of Health cannot be overestimated, and an opportunity for associating the people with the ministry occurs in the Consultative Councils . . . by the creation of a people's council, of which at least half the members should be women and of which a woman should be chairman, any fear that the medical profession in the cause of science, or that government and local officials in their zeal for administration, may overlook the human side of health questions, would, as far as possible, be prevented. (*The Times*, 5 March 1919)

To which Millicent Fawcett replied:

> We have read with great interest Miss Llewellyn Davies' letter in your issue today, and whilst agreeing with much that she says, we would go one step further. We are fully alive to the necessity of securing the closest possible co-operation between the public and the Ministry of Health . . . in our view no more effective means could be adopted to achieve this result than the setting up of a Women's Consultative Council alongside the other councils which it is proposed to bring into being. Responsibility for the health of the nation rests so largely with its wives and mothers that any ministry which hopes to achieve success must take them into close council. [Signed] Millicent Garrett Fawcett, Rosamund Smith, Dorothea Irving, Maud Selbourne, Lady Rhondda. (*The Times*, 6 March 1919, p.6)

The outcome of this episode was better for some than for others.[59] The Ministry of Health was created in 1919. The experts took up the senior positions, and the General Consultative Council (the body which conveyed public opinion) very quickly disappeared, even from an early account of the creation of the Ministry.[52] In particular, women's voices were lost: all of the senior positions went to men, with the exception of Dr Janet Campbell, who took a place at the Ministry with special interest in child welfare. Most poignantly, given the stimulus provided by concern for perinatal and maternal death to the creation of the Ministry, maternal mortality increased for the next 30 years.[64,65]

The public campaign for the creation of the Ministry of Health is a minor episode in the history of health provision in Britain. Nevertheless it encapsulates much that is relevant in the relationship between the public and the health profession. It shows the intensified concern for the public – its health, its "health-behaviour" and its opinions – that came to inform medical politics by the early twentieth century; it indicates the sense of importance attached to the possibility of harnessing public opinion within a medico-political campaign; it shows the importance of mother and child health as a locus for public concern[66,67] and the perceived importance of women in translating health policy in the domestic sphere; it shows the desire of the medical profession to bring to an end the vestiges of lay control of medicine, and the link between this ambition and the emerging Ministry of Health.

PUBLIC INVOLVEMENT IN THE 1920s AND 1930s

There are few accounts of the role of the public in relation to health services in the second and third decade of the twentieth century. By the 1930s, it would appear that the relationship between public and profession was more settled.[54,68] The report published by Political and Economic Planning (PEP),[69] and the series of articles on the nation's health in *The Times*[70] appear to reflect a growing consensus about the value of modern medicine and the desirability of some form of state regulation of health services. It was perhaps because of the consensual view of the value of medicine that Carr-Saunders used doctors as an exemplary model in his sympathetic study of the role of professions in a modern society.[71]

On the other hand, a number of health-related pressure groups were active during the depression. Developments at the Ministry of Health suggest that the consensus needed to be actively maintained. A public relations unit was set up in 1933. At first it dealt only with the press, but from 1936 used films to communicate directly with the public. Some evidence of the importance attached to the work of the PR unit can be inferred from the fact that the Minister of Health attended every one of the fortnightly meetings, each occupying an afternoon.[72]

THE PUBLIC AND HEALTH POLICY IN THE NHS

PUBLIC INVOLVEMENT IN THE CREATION OF THE NHS

The appearance, in the middle of the Second World War, of Sir William Beveridge's plan for a welfare state aroused intense public interest. Over 100 000 copies of the plan were sold in the two weeks after publication on 2 December 1942.[73] Throughout the war public opinion was gathered by a number of government organisations – the War Time Social Survey, the Home Office Intelligence Unit – and by non-governmental bodies such as the British Institute of Public Opinion, the forerunner of British Gallup,[74] and Mass Observation, founded in 1937 (see Ref. 75 for an introduction and bibliography).* The report from the police duty room in Grimsby on 4 December 1942 is typical of those submitted to the Home Office:

> The Beveridge Report has been very favourably received by the general public and it already appears obvious that any attempt seriously to oppose these proposals will be regarded by many citizens as an interference in vested interests. It appears to the writer to have aroused interest in persons who do not ordinarily pay much attention to social problems. (Jones,[76] p.44)

Of all the forms of welfare provision that Beveridge proposed, "free" health care was of particular interest to a large section of the

---

*Mass Observation can claim to have carried out the earliest questionnaire-based surveys of patients' experience of hospitals in 1943 (contained in M-O Archive Health Box 1 File F) and open-ended informal interviews of public attitudes to health and the medical system 1943 (Box 1 File M).

population and the degree of interest aroused by the Beveridge Report contrasts sharply with interest in other public issues of the time.[77,78] A survey by the British Institute of Public Opinion (BIPO), made two weeks after publication of the Beveridge Report, found that 88% of respondents believed that doctors and hospital services should be made free of charge.[79]

In the years between the Beveridge Report and the NHS Act of 1946 public interest in health services was not incorporated into the mordant debate between the medical profession, politicians and civil service (for information on the debate, see Ref. 80). A BIPO survey in 1944 indicated that while the public were overwhelmingly in favour of the principles embodied in the Beveridge Report, there was little interest in the exact form which the service should take.[81] Rather than engage in the debate about the implementation of the Beveridge Report the public expressed a strong preference for the principles it embodied through conventional political means. The Common Wealth Party, which favoured full and immediate implementation of the Beveridge Report, scored a series of spectacular by-election successes, and the view has been expressed that Churchill's silence on the subject of the Beveridge Report was decisive in the public's rejection of the Conservatives at the end of the war.[82]

Although the lack of engagement provides evidence of public passivity between the White Paper of 1944 and the NHS Act of 1946,[54] other evidence indicates the sensitivity of politicians and doctors to questions of public involvement in the planning of services. In the negotiations that took place in Cabinet, and between Bevan, the British Medical Association and the Civil Service, Bevan rejected the proposal of more left-wing colleagues for continued local authority control of the health services, which might have provided a forum for local democratic control of services.[12] (Although their motives were not to do with local accountability, the civil service favoured local authority control of state medical services up to the mid-1940s.[83]) Nor would Bevan concede that the NHS work-force (apart from the medical profession) should have any representation on the various boards that were being established to oversee the NHS.

The arrangements served to exclude any vestiges of lay influence in the provision of health services. Bevan, like members of the medical profession,[84] used the pejorative notion of "meddling" to describe aspects of public interest in health matters. He dismissed complaints made by patients:

> If the [complaints] tribunal were called upon to investigate allegations against doctors brought to them by any person at all, the tribunal might become "a source of petty persecution of the profession, because in the field of medicine there are more idiosyncrasies than in any other human activity". (Bevan: National Health Service Bill Standing Committee C, Official Report for 30 May 1946, quoted in Ref. 16)

Of the three parties that shaped the NHS (Bevan, the BMA and the Civil Service) it is the stance taken by Bevan on questions of public participation that appears most in need of explanation. The reason that Bevan failed to encourage "local voices" was due only in part to appeasement of the medical profession. More importantly, he subscribed to a particular set of views about the place of medical services in a state system, which informed the creation of the NHS. First, he believed that centralisation was the key to efficiency and equality in health services. Second, he considered that the route to population health gain lay in securing access to medical services, particularly hospital services. Bevan's achievement came about because he was able to believe that public interest and the interest of the profession were effectively the same on matters of health and health care provision. He would have agreed in effect with Beveridge's view that it was the highest duty of the patient to comply with medical orders.[73] Bevan is rightly commemorated for fabricating the NHS from the myriad of services and the petty conflicting debates of the 1940s. But he also made it possible for the medical profession to finally realise its long-held ambition to free itself from lay control.

The NHS which Bevan brought into being encapsulated a perspective on the role of experts which gave them authority to determine the form of health provision. The founder of the NHS established a set of principles which a priori denied any need for public participation in the formulation of an effective health service, this in a service that was created in the name of the people. Klein has suggested that a service "for the People" must overlook the wishes and demands of the public and of individuals:

> . . . the real justification of the NHS lies precisely in the fact that it does
> not respond readily to consumer demands: that it is a device for
> compelling collective altruism. (Klein,[85] p.158)

Klein's argument, that the NHS is a professionally controlled means
for the equitable distribution of health resources, addresses the
paradox of non-participation by the public in its health service. The
failure of the NHS to affect class differences in morbidity and
mortality suggests that a more "political" explanation of the paradox
might be possible. That the medical profession was willing to
compromise its autonomy by entering into state employment was
made possible by an idealisation of the role of medicine in society. In
practice the profession was seeking to fulfil a vision of freedom from
lay control. The projection of an idealised past onto the late 1940s
played the role of a founding myth which allowed the medical
profession to surrender its autonomy.

While popular enthusiasm for the NHS was in marked contrast to
public fear and rejection of hospitals in the late nineteenth century,[26]
there is considerable evidence to suggest that the benefits that have
accrued following the formation of the NHS have fallen to the
professional groups within the NHS rather than to the public (for
material on this point see Refs 12, 14, 57, 69, 86–91). Comparing
Logan's 1950 survey of social class variations in mortality[92] with
more recent experience it is evident how little an organised health
care system can contribute to crude, but nevertheless important,
measures of public health. Najman provides direct evidence that the
NHS has had almost no effect on age-standardised mortality rates of
the poorest 1% of the population, while the rates for the wealthiest
1% have declined steadily throughout the postwar era.[93]

The medical profession placed itself within a state welfare perspective
to make professional advance. Webster makes the following claim:

> Concessions [to the BMA] were offered on such a massive scale that
> the objectives for which the NHS was created could only be
> imperfectly realised. In practice, the NHS incorporated precisely the
> kinds of inefficiency and inequity which the new system was designed
> to eliminate. The benefits of state investment in health care were

thereby eroded in the interests of pacifying the medical profession, the voluntary lobby, [and] the drug companies. . . . Once control was seized by professional and corporate groups, it was never willingly relaxed. The NHS was therefore diverted into an arena offering major gains for professional and corporate interests.[94]

Radically opposing the view that the NHS was a popular victory, Webster contends that the creation of the NHS represents a victory for professional rather than the public interests: the achievement of new forms of professional dominance rather than the victory of coherence over heterogeneity of service provision.

The formation of the NHS represents, in part at least, the medical profession's final campaign to free itself from accountability to lay bodies, a campaign which began in earnest, Klein argued, with the National Insurance Act of 1911.[17] Whether or not the desire to end lay control in medicine was a principal aim of the medical profession as it negotiated its role in the NHS is open to debate. But in practice, the establishment of the NHS marks an end to traditional forms of lay accountability and scepticism concerning the value of professional health care.

PUBLIC INVOLVEMENT IN HEALTH SERVICE PLANNING

The history of service planning in the NHS might be assumed to include some form of regular recourse to public views when considering policy options. Yet with recent and limited exception those responsible for planning services have not felt the need to consult users or the wider public before decisions are taken. Such a non-observance of public opinion has a long tradition in the NHS. It was assumed by the principal architects of the early NHS that the form which health services should take would emerge quite spontaneously.[54] For a long time, therefore, planners addressed the relatively straightforward but restricted question of the desirable size of the medical establishment and capital facilities, and excluded considerations of the effectiveness of particular treatments or patient requirements.[95]

The idea that beds were the essential currency of health within the

NHS was unchallenged until the late 1960s.[96] Until this time planning consisted largely in arriving at workable solutions to problems posed in the form of (Beds/Unit Population) and (Consultants/Unit Population) for given specialties or disease categories. In the Leeds Regional Hospital Board, such planning

> was entrusted to the Board's medical advisory committees, which were composed mainly of consultants. [Plans were formed] on the basis of the knowledge of their own members, visits to hospitals, evidence from other doctors, and questionnaires completed by HMC [Hospital Management Committee] secretaries. (Ham,[18] p.50)

The epitome of this approach was the Hospital Plan for England and Wales,[97] which formalised the role of large multi-specialty hospitals identified as district general hospitals (DGHs). The concept was developed as a response to pressure from the BMA to renew hospital stock.[98] The idea was not original, however, having been proposed in 1945 in a survey of London hospitals,[99] and later in a Nuffield Provincial Hospital Trust study.[100]

At some point in the 1960s this view of planning ceased to hold. In its original conception the DGH was a group of multi-storey blocks. Architecturally dominating their locality, DGHs were designed according to the need for internal communication and future expansion. Acute beds were provided at about 3.3 per thousand. The original scheme was never wholly abandoned, but was eclipsed in 1965 by a new design, the "best buy" hospital, of which Bury St Edmunds is an example. The best buy design was different in many respects. Physically, it was low-rise; acute beds were provided at a rate of 2 per thousand catchment population; wards were intended to be organised around the concept of patient dependency rather than specialty; the design offered little scope for physical expansion. Most importantly, the best buy hospital was intended to be integrated with community-based services, outpatient clinics and day surgery.[101] Although the target of 3–4 acute beds per 1000 population was reasserted in the late 1960s,[102] the principles upon which large hospitals were based did not predominate thereafter.

The resident population ceased to be a passive denominator of health care planning equations. It became the unit for which "services" (rather than simply beds or doctors) were to be organised. The shift of emphasis from beds to services, and the emergence of community medicine, marks the beginning of a form of caution towards the professional claims of medicine. From the mid-1960s it was no longer always enough, in the minds of planners, simply to make beds or hospital-based medical attention available in order to guarantee proper health care.

The reasons why the change to population-based planning took place are not clear. The altered perception of need involved in the move from DGH to best buy may have come about because of the need to save money. Similarly, population-based planning came about as a result of the experimental move from capital planning to the Planning, Programming, Budgeting System (PPBS) within the DHSS.[103] It may be that that shift was an attempt to overcome a contradiction within the NHS of the 1960s: whilst spending on the NHS was expanding, largely through the hospital building scheme,[97] a number of people were beginning to suggest that the demand for health care would always outstrip available resources, and that demand could even be induced by suppliers. This pessimistic view of the role of medical services – infinite demand – "the iceberg"[104] – was accepted almost without question at the time.[105] As a result hospitals lost their ability to command the central focus of NHS planning, since there appeared to be evidence that their growth would simply result in the demand for treatment to expand. In the 1974 reorganisation the inversion of the planning equation was complete. Instead of the hospital which served a population, the population itself in the form of particular groups now became the base, at least nominally, from which considerations of resource allocation proceeded.[106]

However, the shift of a planning focus towards services and populations does not provide a guaranteed role for public involvement, since considerations of service or population provision can be at least as technical as those of capital planning. It did however provide an opportunity, realised through the re-entry to the NHS of the Medical Officer of Health, now known as the Community Physician, for the NHS to move to a situation where the idea of patients' needs encompassed more than access to beds and doctors.[107] A few attempts to include the public (or in some cases

NHS staff) in the planning of hospital services in the 1970s and early 1980s were made, but without notable success.[108]

"PRIORITIES FOR HEALTH"

The publication of the first explicit priorities for the health service in 1976[106] was made possible by an experiment undertaken by the DHSS in the late 1960s, which involved the substitution of capital budgeting by the Planning, Programming and Budgeting System, usually referred to as Programme Budgeting.[103] The stated reasons for the DHSS publishing its priorities document were fourfold:

1. To emphasise that growth in public expenditure for the NHS was to slow down from 1976 onwards, whilst the need for health care of particular sorts would continue to grow.
2. To emphasise that marginal increases in capital should be selectively applied according to need and not dispersed randomly within the service, and to indicate that the DHSS considered itself central to this process.
3. To highlight areas of past neglect and propose that they should receive relatively more generous funding in the future.
4. To emphasise central interest in effective and efficient use of resources.

The slogan the DHSS chose to cover these varied aims in its document was "to put people before buildings". But there is no sense of wanting to involve the public in planning decisions; the phrase was used to gloss a small shift of resources away from acute services. It was believed within the DHSS that the Priorities report would lay the foundation for more rational planning, according to population needs.[108] However, the hostility of the medical profession and the vagueness of the methods and concepts contained in the Priorities document and its follow-up publication *The way forward*[109] ensured that little progress was made.[85] Indeed, the policy of bringing about a shift in resources from the acute sector through planning ended in 1988 when new guidelines concisely invited health authorities to:

> plan for levels of activity in the acute sector sufficient to meet referred demand by clinically appropriate treatment. (HC(88)43)

Treatment rate targets were specified: 300 coronary artery bypass grafts, 1050 hip replacements, and 1500 cataract operations per million population per year. *Priorities for health* is the precursor to the modern debate about priorities because it acknowledges the limits to growth and competing claims to resources. But it also signifies the last efforts, along with the Resource Allocation Working Party, of a long NHS planning tradition, a system based, however imperfectly, on the vision of a centrally planned state service. During the 1970s and 1980s the planning system has become more fragmented as planning has been devolved outward first to Area Health Authorities, and then District Health Authorities (Health Commissions).

COMMUNITY HEALTH COUNCILS AS PUBLIC REPRESENTATIVES

The first indication that a special body was to be created to represent the public's views to the NHS came in 1971, when Sir Keith Joseph, Conservative Secretary of State for Health and Social Services, published a consultative document on the future of the NHS.[110] The creation of a formal structure to represent the public within the NHS is a significant development, although Community Health Council (CHC) members have always been nominated rather than elected. To understand why CHCs appeared in the 1970s it is helpful to look at the context in which they were created. The 1974 health service reforms separated responsibility for managing the NHS from responsibility for representing the views of the public and consumer. CHCs were intended to fulfil that role. Along with the Health Advisory Service, their creation was part of the response to effective newspaper coverage of the poor conditions in a number of hospitals, principally psychiatric and elderly long-stay.[111]

The envisaged activities of Community Health Councils gave them a wide remit within the NHS. The Health Circular covering their initial role suggested that Area Health Authorities ought to consult Community Health Councils on matters of general provision, effectiveness of service, and of planned developments.[112] CHCs could also initiate contact with health authorities on these matters.

CHCs could monitor the development of joint planning arrangements between health authorities and local authority social service departments, and the implementation by health authorities of national standards and policies. CHCs were invited to take a specific interest in hospital visiting arrangements, waiting times at clinics, waiting lists and patient facilities, and plans to close hospitals. Investigation of complaints by individuals against clinicians fell outside their remit. Broadly speaking, the role of Community Health Councils has not altered since their original formulation. Ham has suggested that there are four types of contact between CHCs and health authorities: negotiation, consultation, public relations and articulation.[113] The actual role played by CHCs is dependent on the approach of the local Health Authority. Most, Ham suggests, conceive of CHCs as essentially consultative bodies. The ability of CHCs to intervene has been restricted since 1991, following the withdrawal of statutory rights to speak at meetings and visit premises.

The shortcomings of Community Health Councils have been rehearsed on many occasions. The submissions to the 1976 Royal Commission on health services by the Institute of Health Service Administrators and District Administrators put the health authority position succinctly – Community Health Councils took up too much of management's time, they were unrepresentative, they failed to carry out background research, and hindered the making of effective decisions.[114] Accompanying this jaundiced view, the actual organisation and resourcing of CHCs have often been unsatisfactory. Their uncertain origin and constitution have condemned them to face the same sorts of problems throughout their existence. Facilities, finance and access to health authorities are generally insufficient. Service providers have never been issued with guidance on how they should work with CHCs. A survey in the mid-1970s indicated that 68% of CHCs were in dispute with their health authority over the meaning of the word consultation.[115] In response to a set of prevailing difficulties, CHCs have developed varying approaches to their tasks. Some have been quite militant; others have adopted the anodyne stance of "patient's friend". A major difficulty for CHC members was their lack of public visibility, due in part to their lack of representativeness.

Despite their limitations, CHCs have sometimes taken the initiative.

They can take the credit for being the first non-research body to carry out patient satisfaction surveys within the NHS, anticipating the work now carried out routinely by NHS trusts. They have also found ways of gathering patient and public opinion about services,[116] and public perceptions about priorities.[117] As well as gathering opinion, there are also occasions when CHCs effectively articulate public opinion. Ham[113] gives the following example: In Weston-super-Mare, following a newspaper article, the CHC organised a public meeting where women attending asked why there was no well-woman clinic in Weston. The health authority informed the CHC that such a service would be uneconomic. As a result of the health authority's response the CHC held a public meeting at which speaker after speaker complained of the current quality of the service. What the women wanted was the opportunity of unhurried consultations with a woman doctor, and a reduction in the number of tranquilliser prescriptions. Following the meeting the health authority re-considered and a number of changes were instituted.

In isolated instances CHCs can be seen mediating between the public and their health professionals. However, the promise of CHCs remains unfulfilled, and they have not been able to organise effectively or articulate a public voice in the NHS. In the era of general management CHCs have not evolved and are perhaps seen by many as obstructive. In any case the internal market of the 1980s implied a new model of public involvement – as consumers – which relegated CHCs to an uncertain future.

MODES OF REPRESENTATION: CITIZENSHIP AND CONSUMERISM

If we accept the conclusion of the first section of this chapter – that the creation of the NHS was, alongside its better known aspects, the endpoint of lay authority in health policy – it follows logically that there should be little role for the public in determining health policy within the NHS, and this appears to be the actual situation.

It is difficult to explain public regard for the NHS on the basis of the achievements of the NHS or the record of public involvement in the organisation of services. In this section it is argued that public regard for the NHS is underpinned by a symbolic relationship, based on an idea of citizenship. Beveridge proposed state provision of health and welfare services on the basis of a view in which the duties of citizenship were integrated with the benefits of health provision.[118] The idea can be traced to early nineteenth-century France and German social insurance. In Britain health reform as a way of articulating the state and its citizens intensified in the twentieth century. The view that the provision of health services plays an important role in stabilizing the modern states is found in many twentieth-century authors. It has been argued that the modern state is grounded in health issues.[119] Marxists maintain that the provision of health services is part of the settlement between labour and capital in the twentieth century.[120,121] Churchill supported health reform after the First World War because he believed it would give the public a stake in the social order. Klein regards the stabilization of the social order as one of the few unequivocal successes of the NHS.[85] For their part, the public have readily subscribed to the idea that the provision of health services is part of the proper role of a modern society. The existence of public health services seems to reveal the existence of a caring society, or at least a society which might care for its citizens during illness. The public consumes the NHS as the symbol of a society that cares.

However, as a way of defining what it is exactly that the public can expect from its health system, citizenship is a weak idea. Citizenship emphasises the right of access to services, and leaves vague the detail of what can be expected. A health system based on citizenship does not exclude the possibility that rationing might exist. Indeed, rationing in the sense of resource limits within the NHS has always been accepted by the public. Why else would it patiently endure the indignities of the system if it did not feel that waiting and queuing, the whole economy of time, was not somehow linked to the common good? The clinician, as distributor and arbitrator of resources, was central to the functioning of a citizenship-based model of resource distribution. In effect the bargain struck between the medical profession and the state at the time the NHS was created was that in return for guaranteed rights of access for the public as citizens, the medical profession should be given considerably enhanced (on this point see Klein and Howlett,[17] pp.37–72) formal and informal powers of "clinical freedom", a term first used by Lord Dawson of Penn in a House of Lords debate of 1943.[122]

The possibility of considering the public as customers of health services first appeared in government policy in a 1979 Conservative Green Paper *Patients first*.[123]* Since 1989 managerialism (in trusts and health authorities) has brought new forces to bear on the relationship between the outside and the inside of the NHS. In seeking to restrict the citizenship model on which the NHS has hitherto been based, managerialism has tried to limit the role of "outsiders" (such as CHCs) to the decision-making process in the name of efficiency and decisiveness. In doing so a role for the public as consumers of NHS products has been created. Examples of consumer initiatives include: patient satisfaction surveys; telephone help lines; the Patient's Charter; and comparative league tables of hospital performance.

Consumerism may be part of the managerial style in the NHS of the 1990s. Yet broadly speaking the public persists in interpreting the NHS as if it were an element of a welfare system, itself a sign of a caring society, or at least a society that might conceivably care for them personally at some point in their lives. It is difficult to accept that consumers can play a significant role in shaping health policy. The history of public involvement shows the NHS to be a system designed to exclude lay participation. From a theoretical point of view there are grounds for doubt, since the prerequisites of health care consumerism do not exist in the NHS: the existence of a market; a range of competing goods; and high-quality information. From a macroeconomic perspective, there are grounds for believing that the organisation of the future NHS will be inimical to the form of health service the public currently prefers.[131] In the United States, where some of the market conditions exist, there is little evidence to support the view that consumers can play a positive or significant role in structuring the market.[132,133]

---

*In the early 1960s Lees and Titmuss became embroiled in a fierce, essentially political, debate over the value of the concept of consumerism in the health field,[124–128] which led to Titmuss' book-length critique of the relevance of market forces to the welfare sector,[129] which subsequently attracted the interest of health economists.[130]

While consumerism is probably too simple a formulation,[134,135] there have clearly been changes in the general manner in which the public has involved itself in its health care in the period of the NHS[135] and with its relations with the doctors that care for them.[136] The more assertive attitude of the public can be seen in a number of areas: first, in the number of complaints about the service made by members of the public, which has grown, and in the public airing of several serious defects in service provision, for which special channels had to be created, including CHCs, the Health Advisory Service and Health Service Commissioner; second, through the formation of groups like the Patients' Association and the College of Health. The College of Health (set up by Lord Young of Dartington, who also founded the Consumers Association) has fostered a consumerist approach to the barriers imposed by waiting lists. Thirdly, the more assertive attitude can be seen as underlying the formation of self-help groups concerned with particular conditions in recent years. While some of these groups are more or less used by the medical profession as fund-raising bodies, others have adopted a more critical role in relation to the care they are given (e.g. benzodiazapine withdrawal groups). This is particularly seen in the area of maternity services, where consumer pressure groups have been responsible for precipitating significant changes in the views of professionals on the appropriateness of technology and hospital facilities in the management of pregnancy and childbirth.[137] The fourth indication of a more assertive public involves a general intensification of interest in health and disease, as seen in the growth of health shops, complementary therapy, and through increased media interest in health.[138]

CONCLUSION

In historical terms the creation of the NHS represents an endpoint to an extended process of securing medicine from the intrusion of lay judgement and control. In working through their strategies, the state and the medical profession have created a public which, although it has gained the right to receive expert health care, has been given little indication that it has anything useful to contribute to questions of provision or organisation. In essence, the history of the NHS has encouraged the development of implicit priority setting controlled by medical professionals dealing with patients on the basis of individualistic ethics (see Chapter 4). The concept of explicit priority setting in which the public could be involved was therefore an alien one. Thus although in the "old" NHS there was little foundation to support a bargaining structure involving the public, the reorganisation has provided the opportunity for its development. The challenge, however, lies in obtaining real commitment to full pluralistic bargaining.

REFERENCES

1. Higgs E. Disease, febrile poisons, and statistics: the census as a medical survey, 1841–1911. *Soc Hist Med* 1991; **4**: 465–78.
2. Green BS. *Knowing the poor: a case study in textual reality construction.* Routledge Kegan Paul, London, 1983.
3. Winter A. The island of mesmeria. The politics of mesmerism in early Victorian Britain [Dissertation]. University of Cambridge, 1993.
4. Porter R. Quackery and the eighteenth century medical market. In: Cooter R, ed. *Studies in the history of alternative medicine.* Macmillan, London, 1988: 7–9.
5. Granshaw L. The hospital. In: Bynum WF, Porter R, eds. *Companion encyclopaedia to the history of medicine. Vol 2.* Routledge, London, 1994: 1180–203.
6. Peterson MJ. *The medical profession in mid-Victorian London.* University of California Press, Berkeley, 1978.
7. Porter R, ed. *Patients and practitioners. Lay perceptions of medicine in pre-industrial society.* Cambridge University Press, Cambridge, 1985.
8. Lawrence CJ. *Medicine in the making of modern Britain, 1700–1920.* Routledge, London, 1994.
9. Harrison JFC. Early Victorian radicals and the medical fringe. In: Bynum WF, Porter R, eds. *Medical fringe and medical orthodoxy.* Croom Helm, London, 1987.
10. Walters V. *Class inequality and health care: the origins and impact of the National Health Service.* Croom Helm, London, 1980.
11. Lindsey A. *Socialized medicine in England and Wales: the National Health Service 1948–1961.* University of North Carolina Press, Chapel Hill, 1962.
12. Webster C. *The health services since the war. Volume 1: problems of health care – the National Health Service before 1957.* HMSO, London, 1988.

13. Pater JE. *The making of the National Health Service*. King Edward's Hospital Fund for London, London, 1981.
14. Eckstein H. *The English health service: its origins, structure and achievements*. Harvard, Cambridge, MA, 1959.
15. Jacobs LR. *The health of nations: public opinion and the making of American and British health policy*. Cornell University Press, Ithaca, 1993.
16 Maxwell R. *Patient participation in the NHS*. Kings Fund, London, 1988.
17. Klein R, Howlett A. *Complaints against doctors: a study in professional accountability*. Charles Knight, London, 1972.
18. Ham C. *Policy making in the National Health Service. A case study of the Leeds Regional Hospital Board*. Macmillan, London, 1981.
19. Hunter DJ. *Coping with uncertainty: policy and politics in the National Health Service*. Research Studies Press, Chichester, 1980.
20. Arnstein S. A ladder of citizen participation. *J Am Inst Planners* 1969; **35**: 216–24.
21. Marks HM. *Representative health planning: who represents whom?* Harvard School of Public Health, Boston, 1979.
22. Porter R. Lay medical knowledge in the eighteenth century: the evidence of the Gentleman's Magazine. *Med Hist* 1985; **29**: 138–68.
23. Fissell ME. The disappearance of the patient's narrative and the invention of hospital medicine. In: French R, Wear A, eds. *British medicine in an age of reform*. Routledge Kegan Paul, London, 1991: 92–109.
24. Jewson N. The disappearance of the sick man from medical cosmology 1770–1870. *Sociology* 1976; **10**: 225–44.
25. Digby A. *Making a medical living: doctors and patients in the English market for medicine, 1720–1911*. Cambridge University Press, Cambridge, 1994.
26. Hardy A. *The epidemic streets*. Oxford University Press, Oxford, 1993.
27. Richardson R. *Death, dissection and the destitute*. Routledge Kegan Paul, London, 1988.
28. Sigsworth M, Worboys M. The public's view of public health in mid-Victorian Britain. *Urban Hist* 1994; **21**: 237–50.
29. Bynum WF, Porter R, eds. *Medical fringe and medical orthodoxy*. Croom Helm, London, 1987.
30. Inkster I. Marginal men: aspects of the social role of the medical community in Sheffield 1790–1850. In: Woodward J, Richards D, eds. *Health care and popular medicine in nineteenth century England*. Croom Helm, London, 1977: 128–63.
31. Porter R. Spreading medical enlightenment: the popularization of medicine in Georgian England and its paradoxes. In: Porter R, ed. *The popularisation of medicine 1650–1850*. Routledge, London, 1992: 215–31.

32. Neve M. Orthodoxy and fringe: medicine in late Georgian Bristol. In: Bynum WF, Porter R, eds. *Medical fringe and medical orthodoxy: 1750–1850*. Croom Helm, London, 1987: 40–55.
33. Loudon I. Medical practitioners, 1750–1850 and the period of medical reform in Great Britain. In: Wear A, ed. *Medicine in society*. Cambridge University Press, Cambridge, 1992: 219–47.
34. Jewson N. Medical knowledge and the patronage system in eighteenth century England. *Sociology* 1974; **8**: 369–85.
35. Wakely T. Editorial. *Lancet* 1831–2; **i**: 2.
36. Perkin H. *The rise of professional society: England since 1880*. Routledge, London, 1989.
37. Shortt SED. Physicians, science and status: issues of professionalisation of Anglo-American medicine in the nineteenth century. *Med Hist* 1983; **27**: 51–68.
38. Jacyna S. Mr Scott's case: a view of London medicine in 1825. In: Porter R, ed. *The popularisation of medicine 1650–1850*. Routledge, London, 1992: 215–31.
39. Harley Warner J. The idea of science in English medicine: the 'decline of science' and the rhetoric of reform, 1815–45. In: French R, Wear A, eds. *British medicine in an age of reform*. Routledge, London, 1991: 136–64.
40. Harley Warner J. The fall and rise of professional mystery. In: Cunningham A, Williams P, eds. *The laboratory revolution in medicine*. Cambridge University Press, Cambridge, 1992: 110–41.
41. Porter R. The gift relation: philanthropy and provincial hospitals in the eighteenth century. In: Grimshaw L, Porter R, eds. *The hospital in history*. Routledge, London, 1989.
42. Andrew D. Two medical charities in eighteenth century London. In: Barry J, Jones C, eds. *Medicine and charity before the welfare state*. Routledge, London, 1991: 82–97.
43. Marland H. Lay and medical conceptions of medical charity during the nineteenth century. In: Barry J, Jones C, eds. *Medicine and charity before the welfare state*. Routledge, London, 1991: 149–71.
44. Howie WB. Complaints and complaint procedures in the eighteenth and early nineteenth century provincial hospitals in England. *Med Hist* 1981; **25**: 345–62.
45. Winter A. Ethereal epidemic: mesmerism and the introduction of inhalational anaesthesia to early Victorian England. *Soc Hist Med* 1991; **4**: 1–27.
46. Foucault M. *The birth of the clinic*. Tavistock Press, London, 1972.
47. Latour B. *The pasteurization of France*. Harvard University Press, Harvard, 1988.

48. Eyler JM. *Victorian social medicine: the ideas and methods of William Farr.* Johns Hopkins University Press, Baltimore, 1979.

49. Rose ME. *The relief of poverty, 1834–1914.* Macmillan, London, 1972.

50. Checkland SG, Checkland EOA, eds. *The poor law report of 1834.* Penguin, Harmondsworth, 1974.

51. Williams P. The laws of health: women, medicine, and sanitary reform, 1850–1890. In: Benjamin M, ed. *Science and sensibility: gender and scientific enquiry 1780–1945.* Basil Blackwell, Oxford, 1991: 60–88.

52. Newsholme A. *The Ministry of Health.* Putnams, London, 1925.

53. Fee E, Porter D. Public health, preventive medicine and professionalization: England and America in the nineteenth century. In: Wear A, ed. *Medicine in society.* Cambridge University Press, Cambridge, 1992: 249–75.

54. Fox DM. *Health policies, health politics: the British and American experience 1911–1965.* Princeton University Press, Princeton, 1986.

55. Gilbert B. *The evolution of National Insurance in Great Britain.* Michael Joseph, London, 1966.

56. Crowther MA. Paupers or patients? Obstacles to professionalization in the Poor Law Medical Services before 1914. *J Hist Med Allied Sci* 1984; **39**: 33–54.

57. Titmuss RM. Health. In: Ginsberg M, ed. *Law and opinion in England in the twentieth century.* Stevens, London, 1959.

58. Green DG. *Working-class patients and the medical establishment. Self-help in Britain from the mid-nineteenth century to 1948.* Gower, Aldershot, 1985.

59. Honigsbaum F. *The struggle for the Ministry of Health, 1914–1919.* Social Administration Research Trust, London, 1970.

60. Addison C. *The health of the people.* University of London Press, London, 1914.

61. Dawson B. Report of the 88th annual representative meeting of the British Medical Association, Cambridge, 1920. *BMJ* 1920; ii(suppl): 18–19.

62. Dawson B. The future of the medical profession. *BMJ* 1917; ii: 23–6.

63. Dawson B. The future of the medical profession (II). *BMJ* 1917; ii: 56–60.

64. Lewis J. *The politics of motherhood: child and maternal welfare in England 1900–1939.* Croom Helm, London, 1980.

65. Loudon I. *Death in childbirth.* Oxford University Press, Oxford, 1992.

66. Dyhouse C. Working class mothers and infant mortality in England, 1895–1914. In: Webster C, ed. *Biology, medicine and society 1840–1940.* Cambridge University Press, Cambridge, 1981.

67. Arnot ML. Infant death, childcare and the state. *Continuity Change*

1994; **9**: 271–311.

68. Lewis J. Providers, 'consumers', the state and the delivery of health-care services in twentieth century Britain. In: Wear A, ed. *Medicine in society: historical essays*. Cambridge University Press, Cambridge, 1992.

69. Political and Economic Planning. *Report on the British health service*. PEP, London, 1937.

70. Various Authors. *The nation's health*. [Reprinted from the National Health number of *The Times*.] The Offices of *The Times*, London, 1937.

71. Carr-Saunders AM, Wilson PA. *The professions*. Oxford University Press, Oxford, 1933.

72. Boon T. *Industrialisation and Health – introductory conference paper*. Science Museum, London, 1995.

73. Beveridge W. *Social insurance and allied services*. HMSO, London, 1942.

74. Gallup G. *The Gallup international public opinion polls, Great Britain, 1937–75*. Random House, New York, 1976.

75. Calder A, Sheridan D, eds *Speak for yourself: a mass-observation anthology, 1937–1949*. Jonathon Cape, London, 1984.

76. Jones H. Beveridge's Trojan horse. *History Today* 1992; **42**(10): 44–9.

77. Lowe R. The second world war, consensus and the foundation of the welfare state. *Twentieth Century British History* 1990; **1**: 152–82.

78. Harris J. G.D.H. Cole's survey of 1942: did British workers want the welfare state? In: Winter JM, ed. *The working class in modern Britain*. Cambridge University Press, Cambridge, 1983.

79. BIPO. *The Beveridge Report and the public*. The Institute, London, 1942.

80. Honigsbaum F. *Health, wealth and happiness*. Routledge, London, 1993.

81. BIPO. *The nation's health*. The Institute, London, 1944.

82. Addison P. *The road to 1945*. Jonathon Cape, London, 1975.

83. Webster C. Local government and health care: the historical perspective. *BMJ* 1995; **310**: 1584–7.

84. Anon. Priorities. [Editorial]. *Lancet* 1951; **i**: 1001–2.

85. Klein R. *The politics of the National Health Service*. Longman, London, 1989: 2.

86. Sturdy S. The political economy of scientific medicine: science, education and the transformation of medical practice in Sheffield, 1890–1922. *Med Hist* 1992; **36**: 125–59.

87. Wakeley C. The golden age of surgery. [Editorial]. *Lancet* 1957; **ii**: 906.

88. Jones G. *Social hygiene in twentieth century Britain*. Croom Helm, London, 1986.

89. Lindsey A. *Socialised medicine in England and Wales: the NHS, 1948–1961*. University of North Carolina Press, Chapel Hill, 1962.

90. Dawson B. *The nation's welfare: the future of the medical profession*. Cassell, London, 1918.

91. Ministry of Health. *An interim report to the Minister of Health by the Consultative Council on Medical and Allied Services. (Dawson Report).* HMSO, London, 1918.

92. Logan WPD. Social class variations in mortality. *Br J Soc Prev Med* 1954; **8**: 128–37.

93. Najman JM. Health and poverty: past, present and prospects for the future. *Soc Sci Med* 1993; **36**: 157–66.

94. Webster C. Conflict and consensus: explaining the British health service. *Twentieth Cent Br Hist* 1990; **1**: 115–51.

95. Frankel SJ, Coast J, Donovan JL. Health care requirements – a framework for progress in priority setting? In: Malek M, ed. *Setting priorities in health care.* John Wiley, Chichester, 1994: 103–15.

96. Anon. *Hospital building in Great Britain.* HMSO, London, 1969.

97. Anon. *A hospital plan for England and Wales.* HMSO, London, 1962.

98. Abel L, Lewin W. Report on hospital building. *BMJ* 1959; **i**(suppl): 109–14.

99. Ministry of Health. *Hospital survey of London and the surrounding area.* HMSO, London, 1945.

100. Nuffield Provincial Hospital Trust. *Studies in the function and design of hospitals.* Oxford University Press, London, 1955.

101. Smith J. Hospital building in the NHS. Ideas and designs I: from Greenwich to best buy. *BMJ* 1984; **289**: 1437–40.

102. Department of Health and Social Security. *The functions of the District General Hospital.* HMSO, London, 1969.

103. Lee K, Mills A. *Policy making and planning in the health sector.* Croom Helm, London, 1982.

104. Last JM. The iceberg – completing the clinical picture in general practice. *Lancet* 1963; **ii**: 28–31.

105. Todd JW. Wasted resources. *Lancet* 1984; **ii**: 1266.

106. Department of Health and Social Security. *Priorities for health and social services in England: a consultative document.* HMSO, London, 1976.

107. Morris JN. *The uses of epidemiology.* Churchill Livingstone, Edinburgh, 1957.

108. Rathwell T. *Strategic planning in the health sector.* Croom Helm, London, 1987.

109. Department of Health and Social Security. *The way forward.* HMSO, London, 1977.

110. Department of Health and Social Security. *National Health Service reorganisation: consultative document.* DHSS, London, 1971.

111. Ingle S, Tether P. *Parliament and health policy: the role of MPs 1970–75.* Gower, London, 1981.

112. Department of Health and Social Security. *Health Circular HRC (74) 7.*

DHSS, London, 1974.
113. Ham C. *Handbook for Community Health Council members*. SAUS, Bristol, 1992: 6.
114. Anon. *Royal Commission on the NHS*. HMSO, London, 1978.
115. Dunford A. Planning for the consumer: the views of Community Health Councils [MA dissertation]. University of Essex, 1977.
116. South and West Regional Health Authority. *CHCs in action: a selection of topics attracting the attention of Community Health Councils in the South and West Region*. South and West Regional Health Authority, Bristol, 1994.
117. Bowling A. What people say about prioritising health services. King's Fund Centre, London, 1993.
118. Harris J. Beveridge's social and political thought. In: Hills J, Ditch J, Glennester H, eds. *Beveridge and social security: an international retrospective*. Clarendon Press, Oxford, 1994.
119. Foucault M. The politics of health in the eighteenth century. In: Gordon C, ed. *Power/knowledge: selected interviews and other writings 1972–1977*. Harvester Press, Brighton, 1980: 166–82.
120. Doyal L. *The political economy of health*. Pluto Press, London, 1981.
121. Navarro V. *Medicine under capitalism*. Prodist, New York, 1976.
122. Hoffenberg R. *Clinical freedom*. Nuffield Provincial Hospital Trust, London, 1987.
123. Secretary of State for Health and Social Security. *Patients first: consultative paper on the structure and management of the National Health Service in England and Wales*. HMSO, London, 1979.
124. Titmuss RM. Ethics and economics of medical care. *Med Care* 1963; **1**: 16–22.
125. Lees DS. *Health through choice: an economic study of the British National Health Service*. Institute of Economic Affairs, London, 1961.
126. Jewkes J, Jewkes S. Ethics and economics of medical care 1. *Med Care* 1963; **1**: 234–6.
127. Lees DS. Ethics and economics of medical care 2. *Med Care* 1963; **1**: 237–40.
128. Titmuss RM. Postscript. In: Titmuss RM, ed. *Commitment to welfare*. 2nd edn. Allen and Unwin, London, 1976.
129. Titmuss RM. *The gift relationship: from human blood to social policy*. Penguin, Harmondsworth, 1970.
130. Cooper MH, Culyer AJ. *The price of blood*. Institute of Economic Affairs, London, 1968.
131. Whynes DK. The NHS internal market: economic aspects of its medium term development. *Int J Health Planning Management* 1993; **8**: 107–22.

132. Mechanic D. Consumer choice among health insurance options. *Health Affairs* 1989; **8**: 138–48.
133. Vladeck B, Goodwin E, Meyers L, Simsi M. Consumers and hospital use: the HCFA "death list". *Health Affairs* 1988; **7**: 122–5.
134. Stacey M. The health care consumer: a sociological misconception. In: Stacey M, ed. *The sociology of the NHS. Sociological Review Monograph 22.* Keele, 1976.
135. Lupton D, Donaldson C, LLoyd P. Caveat emptor or blissful ignorance? – patients and the consumerist ethos. *Soc Sci Med* 1991; **33**: 559–68.
136. Armstrong D. The doctor–patient relationship 1930–1980. In: Wright P, Treacher A, eds. *The problem of medical knowledge: examining the social construction of medicine.* Edinburgh University Press, Edinburgh, 1982.
137. Jennett B. *High technology medicine. Benefits and burdens.* Oxford University Press, Oxford, 1986.
138. Karpf A. *Doctoring the media: the reporting of health and medicine.* Routledge Kegan Paul, London, 1988.

CHAPTER EIGHT

JENNY DONOVAN AND JOANNA COAST

Public Participation in Priority Setting: Commitment or Illusion?

The previous chapter has shown that lay control of health care has gradually reduced since the nineteenth century, but since the late 1980s there has been an apparent shift towards bringing the public back into the NHS. Initially, this came from the increasing promotion of the rights of consumers, as outlined in the White Paper, *Working for patients* (1989)[1] and revealed more fully in *The Patient's Charter* (1992).[2] The publication of *Local Voices* (also in 1992),[3] an NHS Management Executive document which sought to explain a policy of incorporating public views into decision-making within the NHS, marked a further shift of emphasis. In this document, it was not only the voice of the consumer that was to be heard, but also the views and opinions of local people – the great British public:

> Local people's views should be used . . . to help establish priorities.
> (Local Voices,[3] p.38)

Further, the NHS Management Executive has attempted to make things easier for those planning public participation by providing a set of documents describing the range of methodologies that could be used to obtain public views.[4-6]

By 1995, this apparent commitment had not diminished, with the

Priority Setting: The Health Care Debate.
Edited by J. Coast, J. Donovan and S. Frankel.   © 1996 John Wiley & Sons Ltd.

Government reiterating:

> The Government is firmly of the view that the public should be fully involved in decisions about their own health. (Government response to the first report from the Health Committee Session 1994–5,[7] p.16)

Many health authorities in the UK have responded to the policy by attempting to put phase one into action – obtaining public views – with varying levels of success and satisfaction. The vast majority, however, have not yet chosen to involve the public in phase two – setting priorities or making choices about what health services should be provided.[8] Although there has been enthusiasm for the notion of allowing the public a voice in the decisions about which health services to provide, there has also been dissension.[9] Indeed, a recent report by the Parliamentary Health Select Committee has recommended a "re-think" of the policy of involving the public in setting priorities.[8] The Committee's report lists a number of the difficulties and questions concerning the acquisition of public preferences, and it also states that there is a need both for more research and to be more realistic about what can be achieved.[8]

It would appear, therefore, that the debate concerning public involvement in the NHS is beginning to return to many of the issues skipped over in the rush to implement the hollow policy described in *Local Voices*. The primary aim of this chapter is to concentrate on these somewhat neglected issues, which concern why and whether the public should be involved in decisions about health care, who could and should be consulted, what sorts of views should be included, how they should be collected, and when and how public views and preferences could or should be incorporated into the decision-making structure. Running through these debates is the essential tension, even conflict, raised by the politics inherent in the ultimate aim of the exercise – involving the public in priority setting – and particularly whether there exists real commitment to public participation or if it remains an illusion.

INVOLVING THE PUBLIC: WHY?

The argument for involving the public in health care decision-making in the UK stems largely from the fact that the NHS is a publicly funded service and, as such, should be answerable to its actual and potential consumers. Further (and this also applies to countries other than the UK), with increasing health care costs and restrained budgets, purchasers of health care are facing difficult decisions concerning health care delivery, in that it may not be possible to provide care for all patients in all circumstances. In many cases, these decisions are difficult and often involve issues of equity, in that choices may focus on particular treatments that may be withheld from specific individuals. Increasingly, there is concern that such decisions should become more explicit and open to public scrutiny. In part this is because patients and members of the public are becoming more knowledgeable about health care and more demanding of it. At the same time, health care purchasers feel increasingly exposed as they are responsible for many of the decisions about the allocation of resources for local health services. These factors have converged to form a climate in which, theoretically at least, the contribution of the public is seen to be essential.

There are a number of arguments put forward for *not* allowing the public a say in health care decisions. Some would argue that it is unacceptable for the public to make judgements between, for example, the old and young, deserving and not (however defined). It can be claimed that such choices tap prejudices and preconceptions, even though this is probably just as likely to be the case with implicit rationing by clinicians. It can also be argued that encouraging the public to make such decisions allows health care purchasers to abrogate their responsibilities. It can be argued that health authorities were created to ensure the efficient and effective delivery of health care, and should be able to make informed decisions based on available evidence without needing to consult the public. Where decisions are not controversial, it is likely that the views of the public could be incorporated without difficulty, but in many cases, these decisions are controversial, even unpalatable.

Another, rather different, argument against the involvement of the public arises from the view that the status quo represents rationing by equity and that empowering the public (more particularly patients) could upset this balance.[10] It is suggested that consumer-led demand might lead to a maximising of health for some individuals, and that this is unlikely to be in the best interests of the community as a whole.[10] In an extension of this argument, Klein also indicates that, although advocating public participation appears to be anti-elitist, participation itself is often a very elitist activity which empowers further those who already have most resources at their disposal.[10] This latter point is borne out by a Canadian study in which the random sample of people in the community agreeing to participate in discussions about priority setting had higher levels of education than average[11] (see also below).

The question of whether or not the public should be consulted about setting priorities in health care also raises the further question of the reasons *why* it should be included. If the issues were not difficult and unpleasant, it seems unlikely that the public would have been invited to contribute. The NHS survived until the 1980s without any attempt to include the views of the public, except through parliamentary candidates (via legislation) or the Community Health Councils (CHCs). Health authorities are being strongly encouraged by the government to introduce public consultation in the UK, but it is difficult to assess the real reasons behind this policy. There are further questions about the commitment of health authorities to incorporate public preferences which might differ considerably from what they feel to be in the best interests of the health authority or the general population. Health policy will continue to be made at a national level, with target-led programmes such as the Health of the Nation. At a local scale, public preferences may, at times, directly contradict national policy. It is not clear what health authorities should or would do then – argue for national policies, or implement local preferences?

WHOSE PREFERENCES: WHAT IS/WHO ARE "THE PUBLIC"?

Once the decision has been made to include public preferences, the question of *whose* preferences becomes crucial. It is here that a proper definition of the public is essential. Exhortations to consider the views of "the public" or "local people" conceal a plethora of issues concerning who should or could be included or consulted.

Inevitably, the inclusion or exclusion of some groups or individuals could have significant effects on the content and tone of the opinions expressed.

A variety of forms of "the public" could be asked to inform priority setting, ranging from the total population (citizens) or a sample of this, to specified community representatives (such as councillors, GPs, shop-owners), or consumers (patients). It is clear that some individuals and groups will have strong and particular views about health services. These include those involved in health care provision, such as doctors, paramedics; purchasers; representatives or groups with a special interest in a disease or service, such as charities; patients or users/consumers; and politicians. The influence of each of these groups or individuals can vary according to the particular issue and their position in relation to the decision-maker. Individual consultants, for example, can sway public opinion by identifying and publicising a case with great emotional impact (so-called "shroud-wavers"). Other influential parts of the public with their own particular agendas include pressure groups (such as the Community Health Councils or self-help groups organised around particular illnesses), patients (as consumers, users or complainants), commercial interests (such as drug companies), and the media (in informing generally and publicising specific issues).

Public views and preferences are likely to be influenced by the campaigns of special interest groups, individuals, or the media in general. It will be difficult to assess the effect of such campaigns on members of the selected public. Further, there are many "silent voices" – members or groups within the general public who do not want to make their opinions known, or who are prevented from so doing by the experience or perception of factors such as racism, sexism and so on.

All these different groups are likely to bring different views and preferences to the bargaining table, and it is highly likely that the composition of "the public" that is included in any priority-setting exercise will influence the outcome. There are also important questions to be asked, not only about who should be chosen, but also about how different groups can be included and the willingness of individuals and groups to participate.

WHO SHOULD BE CHOSEN?

There are no available theories that describe which groups should be involved in the process of setting priorities for health care. Value judgements must be made about who should, or should not, be included. In turn, there is a question about who should make these decisions. Again there is no available theoretical basis. It may be, however, that empirical work can inform these decisions.

Research on this issue in the UK has been limited. A survey of the public conducted in Bath found that, while 65% of those questioned felt that "the public should have more of a say in making the decisions", 58% felt that "decisions should be left to the doctors and other experts at the health authority".[12] In City and Hackney, 67% agreed or strongly agreed that the public should have more of a say in making decisions.[13] More detailed work has recently been completed in Canada.[11] This involved asking various groups about their preferences for who should be included in the process of health care decision-making,[11] examining the opinions of randomly selected citizens ($n = 46$), town hall meeting attendees/"interested citizens" ($n = 46$), District Health Council appointees ($n = 61$), elected officials ($n = 38$), and health care and social services experts ($n = 89$). Each group was asked who should be responsible for making decisions.

Overwhelmingly, there was a preference for a combined decision-making body. Participating individuals were asked which groups they favoured being included in a body aimed purely at making planning and priority-setting decisions. A rank order of the results showed that elected officials were considered most important, followed by (in order of importance) the provincial government, experts, DHC appointees, interested citizens and random samples of citizens.[11] These results could, however, have been influenced by the relative proportions of individuals in the different groups. It is of note that in the group of "interested citizens", 77.3% felt that they should have a consulting role in priority-setting decisions and 22.7% felt that they should have responsibility for these decisions. In the group of randomly selected citizens only 47.8% felt that they should have a consulting role in such decisions, with a further 39.1% favouring a role with responsibility. There appears, therefore, to be a strong feeling among interested citizens that they should play a role in these decisions.[11]

As the authors state, there is no reason to think that these results would necessarily be replicated in other cultures and societies.[11] Canadian society and health services are different in many ways from other communities, and so it would be necessary to repeat the study to inform priority setting in other countries. It is of note, however, that even within this one cultural context, the authors conclude that although there are significant differences in the views held by different groups about who should be involved in the devolved decision-making – including priority setting – all groups were overwhelmingly in favour of a combined decision-making body of some sort, giving support to the idea of pluralistic bargaining.

CAN VIEWS BE REPRESENTATIVE?

The desire of particular individuals to be involved in the priority-setting process may not be the only important issue for consideration, however. The inclusion of particular groups and individuals may have specific benefits, but it may also cause the preferences to be biased in particular ways.

Balancing the views of different individuals and groups is a complex matter. It may be, for example, that purchasers of health care incline towards listening to the views of those who most closely represent their own views or those of the status quo. They might also prefer to rely on agents who will act in the best interests of the overall population or of patients. But this is not as clear cut as it seems. Public health physicians, for example, could be seen to be the "champions of the people", as it is their job to have an overall view of the health of the public, and, by implication, to know what health programmes should or should not be in the interest of local or national populations. In fact, they are likely to express the preferences and priorities that reflect their training in traditional biomedicine. It is also the case that many public health physicians are also involved in purchasing, and this may cause some conflict in their role. They may consciously or inadvertently reflect the policies of purchasers in their attempts to obtain public preferences, perhaps through their selection of particular individuals or groups to "represent" the public, or, perhaps more likely, by excluding those who might offer an alternative viewpoint from that of purchasers. Their commitment, then, to obtaining dissenting views from the public may be questionable.

Others who might have a claim to represent the public in some way include Community Health Councils (CHCs) and elected leaders. CHCs often claim to be people's or patients' representatives, but members are not elected but appointed by local authorities, local voluntary groups and health authorities, and so are not likely to be representative in any statistical or intuitive sense. Even elected leaders, such as councillors or MPs, are unlikely to have been elected on their views about the health service, let alone its priorities. They are also likely to express the views of their party on health issues, and, even with wide consultation, will not be able to express the opinions of all their constituents.

The "public" may also be selected at random from published lists. Although this may introduce bias as all published lists have flaws and omissions, the resultant sample, if drawn correctly, should be representative of a local population. It has been suggested, however, that this population should not include those who have recently suffered from a condition involved in the priority-setting exercise as these individuals have too personal an interest.[14] Excluding these particular individuals may, however, rob the priority-setting exercise of important experience. It also raises the thorny question of what other personal (or family) experience of illness should exclude particular individuals or groups.

Another suggestion has been to incorporate the average preferences for particular outcomes of the whole population.[14] It is further suggested by Hadorn that any individual's preferences could then be estimated by reference to an average of "similar" people.[14] Such people could be matched according to a number of criteria, including, for example, demographic characteristics. It is conceded that this procedure would lead to the removal of idiosyncratic preferences, and that it might be challenged on the grounds of stereotyping particular groups. Hadorn suggests, however, that groups could be checked for validity by testing on subjects not included in the original procedure for acquiring the groups, and that the argument about stereotyping cannot be made unless the procedure produces stereotypes.[14]

The issue of who defines the part of the public that will be included in the priority-setting exercise is crucial and influential. The public comprises a wide range of individuals, some of whom form particular groups. These individuals and groups have different backgrounds and experiences, and it is likely that they express a number of contradictory views. If it were possible to sample all the views and preferences of the public, even on an isolated issue associated with priority setting, making sense of the resultant confusion would be arduous. Obtaining a complete and true representation of the public is probably an illusory goal. The form of the public which participates in priority setting can only be partial and to obtain fuller coverage of the many voices available probably requires multiple sampling strategies.

WILLINGNESS TO PARTICIPATE IN PRIORITY SETTING

In 1984, Klein stated that "we cannot start with the assumption that there is a dammed-up demand for greater participation, only waiting for the institutional changes needed to open the floodgates of public involvement" (Klein,[10] p.23). This is equally true in 1995. As indicated above, the subsample of the population that is willing to participate in priority setting is unlikely to be a reflection of the public as a whole. Klein expresses concern both that those groups which are most vulnerable, such as the elderly, are the least likely to be able to assert their own self-interest, and that those most deprived in terms of health care, such as the unskilled and poorly educated, are among the least likely to participate.[10] There is, then, an apparent inverse law of participation, where those in the greatest need to further their interests have the least capacity to do so.[10]

This concern has been borne out by the characteristics of participants in a number of studies, including the Oregon plan.[15] The work by Abelson et al[11] (see above) explicitly aimed to obtain the views of those who, in reality, would be most likely to participate in health care decision-making. They thus aimed to find motivated individuals in all groups but attempted a random sample of the general public. It is clear that even this latter group was very selective, with a response rate of 6% and higher than average levels of education in the responders.[11] The high level of willingness of this group to participate in decision-making, therefore, may not be reflected in the community more generally.[11] The authors of this study concluded that there are significant differences across both groups and individuals in the extent to which they are willing to participate in health care decision-making.

It is also the case that individuals who become involved in an exercise such as priority setting become inculcated into the process, thereby losing some of their ability to participate as an "ordinary member of the public". In particular, when presented with forceful arguments from clinicians or hospital managers, individuals may find it difficult to defend their original views and therefore move closer to the medical viewpoint.

Thus any priority-setting exercise which has included the public needs to be scrutinised with some care. Clearly, there are many different interpretations of which individuals and groups could be considered to fall under the general heading of "the public". Further, even when these are clearly specified, it is still likely to be difficult to assess the representativeness of the individuals and groups selected. The large number of decisions inherent in defining and delimiting the public will clearly influence the priority-setting exercise. Those establishing priority-setting exercises will need to be explicit about their reasons for including or excluding certain groups or individuals if they wish to avoid being accused of "fixing" the result. Further, as obtaining a full representation of the public may be illusory, the partiality of the views obtained will need to be taken into account.

OBTAINING PUBLIC PREFERENCES FOR PRIORITY SETTING: WHAT AND HOW?

Public preferences can incorporate a wide range of attributes, including beliefs, utilities, choices, attitudes, priorities, complaints and views. These may be general or specific, and may be obtained from a number of different individuals and/or groups via several methodologies. The sorts of public preferences that may be collected range from the very specific views of particular individuals (such as complaining patients), to the lay beliefs of local people.

WHAT SHOULD BE ELICITED

At the simplest level, it may be possible to make use of the criticisms that individual patients make of services. Such criticisms may include formal and informal complaints, usually directed at particular service providers or organisational matters by disgruntled patients. Such complaints may be a useful trigger to change, but they are likely to be extreme and represent only the "tip of the iceberg" in terms of general patient views. Any reliance on complaints alone would ignore the views of the majority of the population, both sick and well, and would be difficult to use in isolation for the purpose of setting priorities.

Attitudes and views about priorities can be collected from individuals and groups by methods including questionnaires, public meetings and others (see below). These may include wide-ranging attitudes, such as the preference for acute rather than chronic care; or more explicit priorities, for example that those with a history of alcohol abuse should or should not receive certain treatments. It is difficult, however, to see how such attitudes could be incorporated easily into priority setting unless the issues are very clearly defined before the attitudes are elicited. While the approach of asking members of the local population directly about their attitudes towards explicit priorities may seem to be the most obvious method of obtaining local preferences, there are particular problems. Those questioned may, for example, lack specific knowledge about particular conditions or treatments, and the amount of information they are given is likely to affect their response. It is also the case that discovering people's priorities is only part of the story. The reasons for their attitudes are likely to remain hidden from an exercise directed at explicit priorities, and so health authorities may be faced with sets of conflicting preferences, but with no information about how these have arisen, or how they might be explained or changed.

A much wider view of public preferences would take into account the lay beliefs of local people. These beliefs include common sense, but also incorporate the theories and explanations that ordinary people develop to cope with everyday life, and particularly events that disrupt it, including illness. Lay beliefs underpin views and attitudes as well as much health-related behaviour. It is well known, for example, that consulting a doctor typically occurs only after an individual has tried other courses of action.[16,17]

There is a small but increasing body of academic research devoted to lay beliefs. While much of this has focused on particular groups or medical settings (see, for example, Cowie,[18] Locker,[19] Anderson and Bury,[20] Donovan[21]), there has been a move towards studying members of the general population (see, for example, Calnan,[22] Eyles and Donovan[23]). This work has shown that lay beliefs have developed over many years of experience. They may include "folk" remedies, often handed down through generations and developed through trial and error. Beliefs can include scientific theories, such as the concepts of viruses and modes of infection, as well as common sense ideas. People are able to hold different sets of beliefs in different circumstances, and while lay beliefs are usually internally consistent, they can be conflicting. People may, for example, express clearly the notion that smoking is injurious to health, while also declaring their need to smoke to calm nerves or even to help a chesty cough.[23]

Eliciting lay beliefs is not easy. The uncovering of deeply held beliefs takes time, and usually requires a researcher to interview a small number of respondents in great detail, often on more than one occasion. Large-scale investigations of lay beliefs are thus unlikely to be undertaken as part of the priority-setting exercise. It is the case, however, that a knowledge of lay beliefs can help in the understanding of the particular attitudes and behaviours of individuals and groups. It is important to take an interest in these beliefs in any case, but they may be particularly enlightening where unexpected or apparently inexplicable views emerge from other sources, such as surveys or public meetings.

METHODS FOR OBTAINING PUBLIC VIEWS AND PREFERENCES

There are a number of methodologies that can be utilised on their own or in combination to obtain public views and preferences for use in priority setting. The choice of methodology will depend largely upon the aims of the exercise, and particularly the individuals or groups from whom the preferences are being collected. Methodologies can be quantitative, qualitative, or a combination of the two. Quantitative methods are characterised by their systematic measurement of variables from large numbers of subjects. Data are obtained from a sample of individuals (usually selected at random) in order to generalise about groups following statistical analyses. Quantitative methods are appropriate when there is a recognised need for measures of the incidence and prevalence of characteristics and their relationships, when a structured instrument can be designed, and respondents are able and willing to provide information.[4]

Qualitative methods typically involve smaller numbers of individuals. They allow a much more detailed exploration of issues, and can be particularly useful for uncovering views about sensitive issues or the opinions of disadvantaged or otherwise "silent" individuals or groups. Qualitative methods are most appropriate when information is required about the meanings of, and reasons for, particular behaviours; issues are sensitive and not amenable to quantification; target groups require flexible approaches; or issues require preliminary exploration before a quantitative survey can be devised.[4]

Determining the most appropriate methodology specifically for obtaining public views as part of a priority-setting exercise is not easy and only a limited amount of advice is available (see, for example, Refs 5 and 24). A number of methodological problems arise from each of the major methods. For quantitative studies, these include insufficient numbers of subjects, improper sampling and poor questionnaire formulation. In qualitative studies, attention must be paid to sampling and the interpretation of material collected. Details of the most commonly used methodologies to date for obtaining public preferences for the purposes of priority setting are given below.

Surveys of Public Opinion

Perhaps the most commonly used methodology is the quantitative survey. Within this broad term, there are, however, many forms that such surveys can take, depending on what information is being collected (see above). The usual aim for surveys is to obtain information from individuals that can be aggregated to provide data about the whole population, or specific groups within it. Data are collected in a standardised manner, so that the same questions are asked in the same ways of all individuals. Inevitably, this means that questions have to be relatively simple and straightforward. Surveys can be administered in a variety of ways: by post, interviewer, telephone. They can include whole populations, such as the census, or a sample of identified individuals. The sample itself may be selected in several different ways, depending on the aims of the exercise.

The most commonly used method of sampling is to identify individuals at random from a published list, such as the electoral roll or FHSA register in the UK. Individuals may also be chosen from lists according to a pattern – every nth person, for example – or according to a quota – certain numbers of women aged 55–70, for example. Some surveys include passers-by, or clusters of people in particular localities rather than names from published lists.

Each of these methods has its own problems. Lists may not be comprehensive. Passers-by and clusters in local areas may not be representative of the population. The use of patterns or quotas may introduce significant biases by including or excluding particular groups and/or individuals. Sampling is a complex matter, and a method should be chosen that is appropriate for the questions being asked and the individuals required. Sampling at random from published lists is generally advocated as the "safest" option.

The need to standardise questions restricts the scope of quantitative surveys as questions and possible responses need to be clearly specified. A major problem with surveys is that they are difficult to compare. Each survey that is undertaken tends to have questions designed specifically for it. As these often vary, and because questions or instruments are rarely validated, comparability with other surveys becomes compromised. Survey designs also require that major decisions are taken about the content of the survey before it commences. Careful piloting is essential if surveyors are to be sure that they are asking the right questions in the optimum format. It is almost impossible to carry out adjustments after the survey has commenced.

Surveys can be administered in different ways, depending on the complexity and length of the questionnaire. Questionnaires may be sent by post, but only if due care has been given to the layout and wording of questions so that they can be easily understood and completed by the subject without assistance. Postal questionnaires have so far been shown to be a useful method for obtaining local opinions and priorities. In New Zealand, for example, a postal questionnaire was developed to enquire about individuals' priorities in health care. The questionnaire accompanied a booklet entitled *The Best of Health* which explained about the need to set priorities in health care,[25] and received approximately 8000 responses.[26]

A number of postal surveys have also been undertaken in the UK. In Coventry, for example, a response rate of 52.4% was achieved for a survey of 1000 homes. The survey aimed to find out about local opinion, particularly with respect to access to hospitals, day surgery, preferred location of outpatient appointments, waiting times and GP services.[27] In East Surrey, a postal survey of 2500 individuals was undertaken to find out about "perceptions of health care priorities",[8] and a response rate of over 70% was achieved. In a questionnaire survey of 1500 individuals in Bath, the response rate was 49.2%.[12] In City and Hackney, a postal survey of a random sample of individuals yielded only 45 completed questionnaires out of 353 "eligible" responders, although interview follow-up eventually achieved a response rate of 78%.[13] Utilities based on a rating scale have also been obtained by postal questionnaire.[28]

It is clear that response rates vary between these different studies. Response rates can be affected by a range of factors, including the simplicity of the questionnaire and the number of reminders sent by researchers. The issue of response rates is, however, an extremely important one, particularly as the principal aim of surveys is to produce findings that are representative of the group selected. The failure of groups of individuals to return forms may invalidate the findings. Using a "highly interventionist strategy", a Solihull postal questionnaire asking respondents to value and rank health states managed to obtain an 80% response rate.[29] Other researchers, however, have suggested that a postal survey is not the method of choice in this area because the response rate is likely to be poor, but also because the issues involved in health service priorities are too complex for postal survey alone.[13]

Questionnaire surveys may, however, also be administered by interviewers. This is inevitably more costly in terms of time and personnel than postal administration, but may be essential for some surveys. Questionnaires that are complex, involving jumping from question to question depending on the response, or requiring prompts, will usually need to be interviewer-administered. Interviewers used in surveys will require training, and some assessment of the inter- and intra-interviewer variability will be necessary. The use of interviewers usually produces a higher response rate than other methods, but care must be taken to assess the characteristics of those who refuse to be interviewed.

Interviewer-administered surveys have been used for obtaining public views. In Cardiff, for example, an interviewer-administered questionnaire was used following a postal survey to find out about public preferences for types of individuals who should receive priority (such as young versus old, married versus single, male versus female).[30] A questionnaire was combined with focus groups in North Derbyshire to find out about women's preferences for maternity care services. The questionnaire used a method described as priority search, in which individuals were asked to express preferences within pairs of options.[31] A study in City and Hackney concluded that an interview survey was "undoubtedly the method of choice" (Bowling,[13] p.60).

Questionnaire surveys may also be administered over the telephone. Again, staff will require training, and an estimate should be made of the inter- and intra-observer variation. Telephone surveys have the advantage that they can be quick, avoid the expense of interviewers travelling to meet respondents, and can be linked to computer systems so that data can be entered at the same time as the call. They may be biased because of the distribution of telephones in the population, or the method of obtaining numbers: published directories may not be up-to-date, and many people are now ex-directory. Telephone surveys, including computer-assisted technology (CAT), may be particularly useful for the follow-up of individuals identified previously by another method. A telephone survey was used to obtain utilities for particular health states in the

Oregon experiment.[15] (For a more detailed description of this survey see Chapter 2.)

The results of surveys commonly take some time to emerge. Surveying is a time-consuming business, and if results are required speedily, a survey is not likely to be the best method. There can be a considerable delay between the collection of data, its analysis and then final presentation.

Quantitative surveys can be used to measure change over time, usually by administering the same basic questionnaire to the same individuals over a given time period, such as six months or one year. This is termed a longitudinal study[5] and can be very powerful in showing change over time. The survey may also be repeated at intervals among similar but independent samples – a "tracking survey".[5]

Quantitative surveys are thus common and, in many cases, useful for obtaining information from large groups of people. This information is, however, by the nature of the survey and its administration, likely to be somewhat simple and superficial. It is also important to note that it is often difficult to assess the validity of the questions asked, and the meanings that the questions have to those answering them. It is also the case that people answering surveys want to present themselves as "good" members of society, and so may give answers which are socially acceptable, but do not necessarily represent their own behaviour (see, for example, Ref. 32). The quality and validity of the results of surveys inevitably rest on the quality of the questionnaire and methodology employed. Unfortunately, many surveys suffer from inadequate planning, weak methodology and poor question design. When they are well designed they can be very powerful in conveying the views of particular groups, although by their very nature they tend to represent "average" aggregated opinions (see below).

Qualitative Methods

The general umbrella of "qualitative research" offers several methods which can be used either as an alternative to quantitative surveys, or in combination with them. The aim of qualitative research is primarily to understand as thoroughly as possible the beliefs and experiences of a group of individuals being studied. The focus is on the meanings of experiences for individuals and the reasons for behaviours. Qualitative research does not seek, for example, to count the numbers of people who have a particular disease, but to examine the meaning the disease has for them and the effects it has on everyday life. Qualitative research also allows the exploration of sensitive issues and deeply held beliefs, and could be used to explain views on, and reasons for, expressed health care priorities.

There are two major methods of research which are commonly used and essentially qualitative.

Participant Observation

Participant observation requires that the researcher observes what is going on while participating in activities. In the fullest sense, a complete participant carries out the research unbeknown to others by becoming totally immersed in the activities of the group. At the other end of the scale, the researcher observes in a much more detached way what is going on. (For a detailed exposition of participant observation, see Spradley.[33]) Data are collected by the researcher, either by making comprehensive notes or by tape-recording events. Participant observation may be particularly useful for the analysis of material emerging from public meetings or focus groups.

In-depth Interviews

In-depth interviews are variously termed intensive or one-to-one interviews, field research, interpretative social science, qualitative or depth interviews, or ethnography. In-depth interviews involve the researcher in talking to individuals (or sometimes groups) about a wide variety of issues surrounding the topic under investigation. In some cases, informants (interviewees) are seen only once,[23] although it is more common for the researcher to build up a relationship with informants over time and with a number of interviews.[21,32] The advantages of interviewing individuals in detail and on more than one occasion include the ability to check or clarify points made, and to develop issues further. A disadvantage is that it reduces the number of informants that can be included in the research.

In-depth interviews are time-consuming. Interviews are rarely short, because of the need to build up a relationship and rapport with the informant. Questions are not predetermined, as in structured surveys. The researcher prepares a checklist of topics to be covered by each informant, but the wording of questions and their order of delivery are determined by the progress of the interview, which becomes very much "a conversation with a purpose" (Sidney and Beatrice Webb, quoted in Ref 34). It is usual to tape-record all the interviews with all the informants so that everything spoken, including the tone and inflection, is available for analysis. All the taped material has to be transcribed, and it takes about five minutes for an experienced typist to transcribe one minute of audio tape.[23] There are thus practical limits to the number of interviews that can be undertaken and analysed.

There are also substantive reasons why the numbers are and should be limited. It is a common criticism of qualitative research that its small numbers cannot mean anything in comparison with quantitative research. In-depth interview research generally involves relatively small numbers, usually of the order of 20 or 30 interviews,[21,32] although sometimes more.[23] A great deal can be said about such groups – each of these pieces of work has produced a book – but what is said is not couched in terms of statistical representativeness, nor should it be. It is not the aim of qualitative research to indicate the quantities of variables within groups of the population – this is more properly the concern of quantified surveys (see above). The aim of qualitative research is to explore and describe in detail the perceptions and experiences of particular individuals or groups *from their point of view*. The intention of in-depth interviews is to try to understand the perspectives of the individuals or groups being interviewed, and to explore the reasons for behaviours, the beliefs that underpin actions, and sensitive issues, all of which are not accessible in a structured survey.

The representativeness of qualitative research is frequently questioned, but sampling for in-depth interviewing is not determined by the need to be representative or to exclude all confounding variables. This is the aim of structured survey work. In qualitative research, the sampling format is largely determined by the nature of the study and pragmatic concerns such as access to, and availability of, informants. In some qualitative studies, for example where in-depth work is required to illuminate and explain the findings of quantitative surveys, it may be possible and desirable to draw a random sample from the electoral roll or other published lists (see, for example, Ref 23).

For the purposes of priority setting, sampling could be random or more purposeful. Glaser and Strauss, for example, suggest "theoretical sampling", in which cases should first be collected to maximise the range of categories generated, and then be selected to test that the categories hold true.[35] Other sampling strategies include the use of a key informant, who gives access to a number of informants; or snowball sampling, in which informants pass the researcher on to others in their social network (see Refs 21, 32, 34).

Sampling may be organised according to time, people or context,[36] depending upon the aim of the exercise. Attitudes and views about health care and priority-setting issues may change over time, between people, and, perhaps most importantly, according to the context in which they occurred or were asked about. Qualitative research techniques allow the exploration of these factors, which may be crucial in understanding the responses of individuals and groups to the priority-setting exercise.

In qualitative research, the emphasis is on understanding the world from the perspective of the informants. Instead of testing predetermined theories (deduction), qualitative research starts from the premise of attempting to understand how the informants view the world, and theory is built up (induction). The analysis of in-depth interviews (and participant observation) requires lengthy and painstaking scrutiny of transcriptions and field notes, which can be aided by computer programs. Ideally, the analysis should proceed concurrently with the interviews. Categories and developing theories can then be challenged and/or substantiated by new material from interviews. Results are typically presented in detail, in the form of lengthy descriptions of the research setting, and the perceptions and experiences of the informants, alongside theoretical insights.

In-depth interviewing techniques are likely to be of relevance to priority setting, which makes use of public preferences in a number of ways. Many of the issues concerned with priorities are sensitive or require thought and/or discussion before an opinion can be reached, and these can be much more easily and successfully collected by in-depth interviews rather than structured postal or interviewer-administered surveys. Further, while surveys may collect information about predetermined categories of preferences or priorities, in-depth interviews can allow the exploration of the reasons for these expressions and views which lie outside those defined by the researcher.

In-depth interviews can be used on their own and in association with other methods, including structured surveys and public meetings. They have been used successfully in the Wirral,[3] and in West Dorset as part of an initiative called PATCH (planned approach to community health), which also makes use of public meetings.[3]

Public Meetings

Public meetings have been used to obtain information about public preferences for priority setting. These have taken two basic forms. Specially convened public meetings focusing on particular aspects of priority setting have been established in Oregon,[15] Bromsgrove and Redditch Health Authority,[3] North Essex Health Authority,[8] and New Zealand.[37,38] Public meetings have also been established with local organisations, such as local employers (e.g. Vermont[39]) or community groups and tenants associations (e.g. City and Hackney Health Authority[13,40]). Public meetings can have a wide variety of aims, but in particular the meetings already conducted have aimed to elicit the priorities for health care held by individuals in a locality.[13,15,40] In one case, this was done by asking individuals to rank various treatments in order of priority ranging from essential to less important.[13,40] In another, the aim was to generate statements about what makes health care important to members of a community, and then these social values were ranked according to the frequency with which they were mentioned.[15]

There are distinct problems associated with the use of meetings as a means of obtaining "public" preferences. The most obvious of these is their lack of representativeness. Meetings convened for particular groups are likely to be subject to volunteer bias, in that it may be only the most informed, or the most concerned, or those members of society with the greatest incentives or fewest constraints who attend. This bias may have a considerable effect on the opinions expressed. The bias may be further compounded by the fact that speakers at public meetings tend to be confident and practised at public speaking. Unless the meeting is very informal, or the issue very emotive, speakers will tend to emerge from particular (typically well educated) groups. The preferences of the individuals attending and speaking at meetings are thus likely to differ considerably from those of the "general" public. Such bias has been noted as a feature of many of these meetings.[13,40,41]

A further problem is that there is no distinct and validated methodology for analysing views expressed at public meetings. A number of different processes have been used thus far, including questionnaires,[40] and counting the frequency of mention of particular issues.[15] Questionnaires may better represent the opinions of the public if administered through random sampling. Ranking of values according to frequency of mention has also been criticised as not generating a credible listing of the health care priorities of the public.[42] Further, the noting of the frequency of issues mentioned requires some a priori definition of the issues, and relies on correct interpretation by the individual noting the responses.

Public meetings may be particularly appropriate in the first instance, where some views are required as a starting point without necessarily having a particular priority-setting model in mind. They may also be used to discuss specific (usually emotive) issues such as the option of closing a local facility. Owing to their high levels of bias, however, it is unlikely that "public" meetings could ever be the sole method for gauging public views.

Other Methods

Other methods are also available, although these have been used less often in priority-setting exercises. These methods include focus groups, health forums, rapid appraisal, community initiatives, patient satisfaction surveys, telephone hotlines/helplines, and consultation with local voluntary groups.

Focus groups are specially convened groups of local people that can be used to assess some aspects of public perceptions and to set the agenda for wider surveys. Groups usually meet only once to discuss a particular issue in some detail, and members may be drawn randomly from the local population or, more typically, from a particular section of the community. In Coventry, four focus groups were used to derive questions which were later used in a questionnaire survey.[3] In North Derbyshire, two attempts have been made to use focus groups. In the first, a market research company recruited a sample of the community from passers-by and the discussions of the groups were taped, transcribed and analysed.[3] Focus groups were also used in combination with a questionnaire survey to obtain information about maternity care.[31] As with public meetings, focus groups are probably not suitable as a sole method of obtaining views and preferences. They can, however, be useful in establishing issues of interest to local people and as preparatory work for questionnaire surveys.

Health forums are similar to focus groups, except that they tend to meet on a regular basis. Health forums are usually locality-based groups drawn from a cross-section of the community, and meet on a regular basis to encourage the development and maintenance of a two-way dialogue between health authorities and local communities.[3] To date, health forums have been used in Bromsgrove and Redditch,[3] Great Yarmouth and Waveney,[3] and by Wirral FHSA.[3]

The *rapid appraisal* method was developed by Ong and colleagues, and uses a combination of public forums and interview survey methods.[43] The aim of rapid appraisal is to gain insight into a community's own perspective on its priority needs, to translate these findings into managerial action, and to establish an on-going relationship between service commissioners, providers and local communities.[5] It can involve eight different stages over a short time period. An important aspect of rapid appraisal is the reliance on community representatives and leaders, such as councillors, teachers and corner shop-owners. Clearly the choice of such "representatives" is crucial.

The aim of a *community initiative* is to develop "locality based approaches to purchasing which involve developing direct links with local people, building up a profile of local needs and agreeing an action plan for meeting those needs with local people" (*Local Voices*,[3] p.10). West Dorset health authority has established PATCH, in which the health authority has been divided into 11 localities, each of which is developing a local profile of health needs, views and service preferences using interviews and forums, with a view to developing an action plan with local people.[3] The initiative is intended to be a two-way process, assisted by the use of facilitators.[3] If ultimately successful, it may prove a model which could be implemented elsewhere. Locality purchasing, based on community initiatives, has been undertaken in Bath, East Sussex, North Yorkshire, South East London and Stockport.[44]

Although *patient satisfaction surveys* are one of the most common methods of seeking patient views about the health service, inevitably it is only the opinions of recent patients that are taken into account, thus limiting their usefulness. Although recent patients have a direct experience of treatment in the National Health Service, they are clearly a biased group. When asked to express priorities, it would be surprising if they did not want priority for their own condition. It is also the case that many patient satisfaction surveys are established without due consideration for sampling and questionnaire development. Patient satisfaction surveys have a tendency to produce the same sorts of findings: that, in general, patients are satisfied with the NHS, but that they have specific complaints about matters such as waiting times, food and decor. They are unlikely to be useful for priority setting.

There are also problems of bias with *telephone hotlines*. People contacting hotlines are likely to be those with the strongest opinions, with fewest constraints to expressing those opinions, and with access to a telephone. The use of a telephone hotline may produce a rapid response to an emotive appeal, but that response is unlikely to be representative of "the public", however defined.

Methods: A Conclusion

There are, thus, very many methodological techniques that may be used to obtain public preferences for use in priority setting. The methodology chosen will be crucial in determining the quality of evidence obtained, and is, therefore, very important. It is not, however, the most important factor to be decided upon early in the process of encouraging public participation in priority setting. There are many more crucial issues that require debate and decisions and which, in turn, will help to define the most appropriate methodology. It is interesting, however, that many of those involved in priority-setting exercises have found it easier to debate methodological minutiae and establish research projects rather than focusing on other influential but difficult issues outlined in this chapter.

SHOULD PREFERENCES BE AGGREGATED?

The necessity for aggregating preferences is likely to depend on the numbers of parties involved in the political bargaining process. If public opinion derived from a number of sources is brought to the bargaining table, there may be divergent opinions. Averaging these opinions will produce a view that is "in the middle" – it will, in all probability, remove any extreme or idiosyncratic opinions. In some cases this may be desirable, but it may also lead to an unnecessary "flattening out" of public opinion. Health and illness are complex matters and people imbue them with a wide range of beliefs and emotions which may fluctuate and even conflict, depending on the issue under consideration. Averaging out the views that people express, for example about different health states, may remove from the priority-setting exercise those things that explain why people act in the ways they do (see Ref 45).

Economists and social policy analysts, in particular, have concentrated on the difficulties associated with making social choices based on individual preferences. Ordinal preferences could be combined in a method akin to voting: if more individuals prefer increased community care (A) to increased acute care (B) then increased community care could be provided. There are, however, problems associated with the use of such voting schemes. For example, assume the choice is now between three options, A, B and C, where C is increased maternity care. It is quite possible that there exists a majority of individuals who prefer A to B, a majority who prefer B to C, and a majority who prefer C to A. Any of the three options could then be chosen depending on how they are presented.*

There are, then, considerable problems associated with the whole question of the aggregation of preferences expressed by individuals. There is no theoretically perfect way in which preferences can be aggregated, and in any case aggregation of preferences may lead to an undesirable averaging of the views of the public. For the practical purposes of priority setting in health care, however, aggregation of preferences may be unavoidable. Unless consensus can be reached, the question of aggregation will have to be faced. In turn, consensus is unlikely unless it is only the views of very small numbers of individuals that are incorporated. The issue of aggregation requires careful consideration, and the method used (such as majority voting, rank-order voting, taking the mean or median preference) will affect the results that are obtained. It may be that preferences will require weighting, as, for example, when certain individuals or groups are perceived to have greater influence than others. If possible, it would be sensible to assess the results using more than one method of aggregation. In some cases, the method of aggregation will be determined by the chosen methodology. In others, however, it will require a choice and it is important that the method of aggregation does not obscure the information obtained from the priority-setting exercise.

INCORPORATING PUBLIC PREFERENCES: WHEN AND AT WHAT LEVEL?

Although purchasers are being increasingly exhorted to make health services more responsive to the needs, views and preferences of local

---

*This problem is known as the paradox of voting and is a specific example of a more general problem, known as Arrow's Impossibility Theorem.[46] Arrow's theorem shows that there is no perfect way to make social choices or to "aggregate" individual preferences to obtain a single social preference.[47] If certain basic conditions, such as non-dictatorship, and the independence of irrelevant alternatives, are to be fulfilled, it is not possible to use individual preferences to derive social preferences.[48] Further information on Arrow's Impossibility Theorem can be found elsewhere.[46–48]

people, and to involve local people in needs assessment, purchasing choices and setting priorities,[3] the level of their commitment to public participation is not easy to determine. An indication of their commitment would be some debate about how, practically, public views will be incorporated into priority-setting exercises and health care decision-making. The questions of when and at what level public views could or should be incorporated into priority setting have, however, received little consideration in the UK.

In many health systems, including the NHS, there is a purchasing cycle during which decisions are made based on some form of implicit or explicit priority setting. Purchasers have a number of choices about when to collect public views, and the point at which they will incorporate them into the purchasing cycle. If the public views accord with their own, then their absorption is likely to be relatively easy. Problems arise, however, when there are clear differences between the public and purchasers, such that, for example, the public desired something that the purchasing authority felt to be completely unacceptable (e.g. no treatment of individuals aged over 70). It is not clear then whether the purchasing authority should follow the public preferences obtained or ignore them.

It may be that some public preferences are included and others ignored, but if only those agreeing with purchasers' views are included, then there would seem to be little point in carrying out the public participation exercise. Commitment to public participation may involve purchasers, for example, entering into a debate with the public over issues involved with effectiveness, equity or efficiency, or producing literature explaining their actions. Such exigencies could require considerable planning and expense.

There is also the question of the level at which the public should be asked to participate in decisions about health care priorities. The public could be asked, for example, whether or not it wishes to participate at all, or whether there should be some other method, be that implicit or explicit. The public could be asked to express general views as to whether priority setting should be based upon particular techniques. It could also be asked more specific questions, for example, about priorities between large clinical areas (such as acute services or mental health), or more defined clinical areas (such as alternative treatments for the same condition), or types of individuals (such as premature babies or the elderly), or closing old or planning new facilities. Again, decisions about the level at which questions are posed will be crucial to the sorts of views elicited and the use to which they can then be put. These issues require considerable debate if there is a real commitment to public participation in priority setting.

PUBLIC PARTICIPATION IN PRIORITY SETTING: COMMITMENT OR ILLUSION?

This chapter has attempted to tackle some of the many confusing and conflicting issues surrounding the involvement of the public in priority setting. There are very many factors that will impinge on the ability of the public to participate in priority setting, and a wide range of decisions that could influence the results. Many of these issues appear to have been neglected in the rush to implement the somewhat vacuous policy outlined by the government since the late 1980s.

It is particularly difficult to assess the level of commitment of government, health authorities and purchasers to the concept of public participation. In part, calls for the public to be involved in decisions about resource allocation have emerged from the development of consumerism (see Chapter 8). It is interesting, however, that this only applies to health care, with little discussion of public involvement in other political arenas such as defence or social services. Perhaps it is an acknowledgement of the increasing interest of members of the public in health care, their familiarity with it from a wide range of media outlets (television, newspapers, magazines, etc.), and a realisation that ordinary people can and should be involved in difficult decisions that are likely to affect their or their families' lives. It may also be that the commitment to involving the public comes from the unwillingness of purchasers to continue to take sole responsibility for difficult decisions about resource allocation.

Whatever the real reasons for the development of the policy for public participation, a strong level of commitment to it is not immediately apparent from published sources concerned with debates in this area or results from priority-setting exercises which are relatively sparse. In particular, the debate has appeared to have become stuck in the rut of describing methodologies for obtaining public preferences, while other issues, such as why the public should be involved, which members of the public should be consulted, what they should be asked, and when and how their views should be incorporated into purchasing decisions, have been somewhat neglected.

Although it is difficult to argue against the platitude that the public should be involved in decisions about health care, it may be that the goal of obtaining and using the preferences and views of the public is an illusory one. The public represents a complex body of opinion, composed of many different groups and individuals producing often divergent views depending on their experiences and perceptions of need. No groups or individuals can easily "represent" the public, even within defined geographical or social areas.

For those wishing to set priorities by employing a technical model, such as equity, the issue of public participation may be irrelevant. It is also likely to be unimportant for those advocating implicit rationing, particularly if this represents the status quo or is controlled by clinicians. It is mainly, although not exclusively, within the concept of pluralistic bargaining that the public, in combination with a range of other groups, can take an active part in setting priorities for health care. It is always going to be the case that the "representatives" of the public (however these are defined) are likely to be the least powerful contributors because of their lack of familiarity with public speaking and limited knowledge of medicine and the workings of the health service. Thus considerable commitment is required by all other groups involved in the exercise, particularly purchasers of health care, if public participation in priority setting is not to remain an unobtainable, illusory goal.

REFERENCES

1. Department of Health. *Working for patients*. HMSO, London, 1989.
2. Anon. The Patient's Charter. *NHSME News* 1991; **50**: 1–2.
3. NHS Management Executive. *Local voices. The views of local people in purchasing for health*. Department of Health, London, 1992.
4. Sykes W, Collins M, Hunter DJ, Popay J, Williams G. *Listening to local*

voices. A guide to research methods. Volume I. Summary of main issues. Nuffield Institute for Health Services Studies, Leeds, and The Public Health Research and Resource Centre, Salford, 1992.

5. Sykes W, Collins M, Hunter DJ, Popay J, Williams G. *Listening to local voices. A guide to research methods. Volume II. An introduction to available research methods.* Nuffield Institute for Health Services Studies, Leeds, and The Public Health Research and Resource Centre, Salford, 1992.

6. Sykes W, Collins M, Hunter DJ, Popay J, Williams G. *Listening to local voices. A guide to research methods. Volume III. The research process.* Nuffield Institute for Health Services Studies, Leeds, and The Public Health Research and Resource Centre, Salford, 1992.

7. Department of Health. *Government response to the first report from the Health Committee session 1994–95.* HMSO, London, 1995.

8. Health Committee. *Priority setting in the NHS: purchasing. Volume 1.* HMSO, London, 1995.

9. Pfeffer N, Pollock AM. Public opinion and the NHS. The unaccountable in pursuit of the uninformed. *BMJ* 1993; **307**: 750–1.

10. Klein R. The politics of participation. In: Maxwell R, Weaver N, eds. *Public participation in health.* King Edward's Hospital Fund for London, London, 1984: 17–32.

11. Abelson J, Lomas J, Eyles J, Birch S, Veenstra G. Does the community want devolved authority? Results from deliberative polling in Ontario. *Can Med Assoc J* 1995; **153**(4): 403–12.

12. Richardson A, Charny M, Hammer-Lloyd S. Public opinion and purchasing. *BMJ* 1992; **304**: 680–2.

13. Bowling A. *What people say about prioritising health services.* King's Fund Centre, London, 1993.

14. Hadorn DC. The role of public values in setting health care priorities. *Soc Sci Med* 1991; **32**(7): 773–81.

15. Oregon Health Services Commission. *Prioritization of Health Services. A report to the Governor and Legislature.* Oregon Health Services Commission, 1991.

16. Kleinman A, Good B, Eisenberg MD. Culture, illness and care. *Ann Intern Med* 1978; **88**: 251–8.

17. Hannay DR. *The symptom iceberg.* Routledge Kegan Paul, London, 1979.

18. Cowie B. The cardiac patient's perception of his heart attack. *Soc Sci Med* 1976; **10**: 87–96.

19. Locker D. *Disability and disadvantage.* Tavistock, London, 1983.

20. Anderson R, Bury M. *Living with chronic illness.* Unwin Hyman, London, 1988.

21. Donovan JL. *"We don't buy sickness, it just comes".* Gower, Aldershot, 1986.

22. Calnan M. *Health and illness.* Tavistock, London, 1987.
23. Eyles J, Donovan JL. *The social effects of health policy: experiences of health and health care in contemporary Britain.* Gower, London, 1990.
24. Donn M. Listen and learn. *Health Service J* 1990; **10 May**: 701.
25. National Advisory Committee on Core Health and Disability Support Services. *The best of health. Deciding on the health services we value most.* Department of Health, Wellington, New Zealand, 1992.
26. National Advisory Committee on Core Health and Disability Support Services. *The best of health 2. How we decide on the health and disability support services we value most.* National Advisory Committee on Core Health and Disability Support Services, Wellington, New Zealand, 1994.
27. Caspe. *Coventry Health Authority survey of future provision of services.* CASPE Ltd, London, 1991.
28. The EuroQol Group. EuroQol© – a new facility for the measurement of health-related quality of life. *Health Policy* 1990; **16**(3): 199–208.
29. Ham C, Honigsbaum F, Thompson D. *Priority setting for health gain.* Department of Health, London, 1993.
30. Vetter N, Lewis P, Farrow S, Charny M. Who would you choose to save? *Health Service J* 1989; **99**: 976–7.
31. Department of Research and Information. *"What kind of maternity care do you want?" Results of a priority search survey of 721 women living in North Derbyshire, November–December 1991.* North Derbyshire Health Authority, Chesterfield, 1992.
32. Cornwell J. *Hard earned lives: accounts of health and illness from East London.* Tavistock, London, 1984.
33. Spradley JP. *Participant observation.* Holt, Rhinehart and Winston, New York, 1980.
34. Burgess R. *Field research: a manual.* Allen and Unwin, London, 1982.
35. Glaser BG, Strauss AL. *The discovery of grounded theory: strategies for qualitative research.* Aldine, Chicago, 1967.
36. Hammersley M, Atkinson P. *Ethnography: principles in practice.* Tavistock, London, 1983.
37. Anon. Public forums – the public's opinion. *The Core Debater* 1994; **3**: 7.
38. Anon. Who should get treatment first – what the public thinks. *The Core Debater* 1995; **4**: 2–4.
39. Bowling A. Setting priorities in health: the Oregon experiment (part 1). *Nurs Stand* 1992; **6**(37): 29–32.
40. Tomlin Z. Their treatment in your hands. *The Guardian* 1992; **29 April**.
41. Klein R. Taking the consumer pulse: are we in danger of overdoing it? *Health Direct* 1992; **March**: 6–7.
42. Dougherty CJ. Setting health care priorities. Oregon's next steps.

Hastings Center Rep 1991; **May–June**: 1–9.

43. Ong BN, Humphris G, Annett H, Rifkin S. Rapid appraisal in an urban setting, an example from the developed world. *Soc Sci Med* 1991; **32**(8): 909–15.
44. Ham C. Local heroes. *Health Service J* 1992; **19 Nov**: 20–1.
45. Donovan JL, Frankel SJ, Eyles JE. Assessing the need for health status measures. *J Epidemiol Commun Health* 1993; **47**(2): 158
46. Arrow KJ. *Social choice and individual values.* Wiley, New York, 1963: 2.
47. Varian HR. Welfare. In: *Intermediate microeconomics. A modern approach.* W W Norton, New York, 1990: 524–36.
48. Ng Y-K. *Welfare Economics. Introduction and development of basic concepts.* Macmillan, London, 1983: 2.

PART FIVE

A Way Forward

CHAPTER NINE

JOANNA COAST

Clarification and Acceptance: A Way Forward in Priority Setting

This book has attempted to clarify many of the areas of confusion surrounding priority setting. This chapter will complete the process by revisiting the conflicts exposed in Chapter 1 in the light of the discussions throughout the remainder of the book. The chapter will, however, look forward as well as back, by charting a course in which the inherent conflicts are accepted and acknowledged. This is the model of health care requirements. It is, of course, only one of many policy options that could be pursued by those setting priorities and it is in no sense perfect. This lack of perfection does not require apology given the impossibility of a "final solution" to the problems exposed by the rationing of health care.

This book is intended to be of practical use, and so the model provided is one which could be utilised at the present time. It does not make heroic assumptions about data availability, nor does it leave the process entirely to clinicians with merely a token input from the public. The model of health care requirements aims to accept the conflicts of priority setting and work within them. By combining technical methodologies with pluralistic bargaining, it both opens up the decision-making process and improves the information upon which priorities are based.

Priority Setting: The Health Care Debate.
Edited by J. Coast, J. Donovan and S. Frankel.   © 1996 John Wiley & Sons Ltd.

Before discussing this model, however, the confusion endemic to the priority-setting debate must be revisited.

CLARIFYING THE CONFUSION

IMPLEMENTATION

This book has attempted to clarify the priority-setting debate by distinguishing between means of developing priorities: technical methodologies versus bargaining processes. It has not concentrated in any great depth upon the issues of implementation, except for a brief comment in Chapter 1. Here, the view was expressed that the implementation of political bargaining approaches may potentially have more support than other means. This support may come about where those involved in bargaining are also those responsible for setting priorities. Where this is not the case, however, implementation may be no simpler than for technical priority-setting approaches.

Other authors have specified the rationing debate, not in terms of the development of priorities, but largely in terms of how these priorities are implemented.[1] Ham has argued that the two main approaches to priority setting are rationing by exclusion, as evidenced by Oregon, and rationing by guidelines, as in New Zealand.[1]

It is contended here that to specify this debate purely in terms of implementation is a mis-specification of the real issues. The major distinction between these two attempts to set priorities is not between their methods of implementation, but in the ways in which they developed their sets of priorities. There is no reason why Oregon's technical priority-setting exercise could not have resulted in a set of guidelines, nor why New Zealand's consensus approaches could not have resulted in a set of exclusions.

This is not to say that implementation is not important. It is vital. But implementation has to do with a great deal more than whether instructions about priorities go out in the form of "fixed" lists or guidelines. It has to do with the incentives faced by those people who will implement priorities. These include not just the incentives faced by clinicians, but also those faced by politicians and managers, and they may include financial incentives as well as those produced by workload, peer pressure and the ballot box. This huge area of research is by no means simple, and is certainly beyond the scope of this book. Hence this chapter will restrict itself, as the rest of the book has done, to the question of developing explicit priorities.

IMPLICIT VERSUS EXPLICIT

The conflict between implicit and explicit rationing was largely dealt with in Chapter 1 and touched upon in Chapters 2, 3 and 4. Following the much-discussed Oregon experiment, there seems to have been a resurgence in the fashion for implicit rationing.[2] It is becoming increasingly difficult, however, to maintain the pretence that there is no rationing. As information becomes increasingly available to patients they are more likely to challenge the decisions made for them by doctors.[2,3] The great attentiveness of the media to the few cases where rationing is acknowledged[4,5] also contributes to a climate in which it is hard to delude the population with the notion that everything desired can be provided.

As in Chapter 1, the remainder of this chapter assumes that implicit rationing – rationing which is not clearly expressed or acknowledged – is not the way forward.

TECHNICAL METHODOLOGIES VERSUS PLURALISTIC BARGAINING

Throughout this book a distinction has been made between setting priorities using technical and political methods. In Chapter 2 the priority-setting attempts of Oregon and New Zealand were examined and it was concluded that, although each employed both options to some extent, the Oregon experiment was more heavily weighted towards methodological techniques and the core services approach of New Zealand was based mainly on pluralistic bargaining. Both options have therefore been used in practice –

despite the legion of criticism that can be applied to each approach. It is not true, therefore, for either approach, to say that it is impossible.

It would, however, be unrealistic to expect to apply technical methods to priority setting at all levels and in all areas of health care with any degree of accuracy or quality. Such a policy would be both too complex and too costly. The experience of Oregon underlines this point. The "guesstimates" used in developing the plan have made commentators wary about the precise nature of the priorities developed and critical of the plan in general.[6–8]

There are, however, concerns about the value of applying a political bargaining approach with no attempt either to provide a framework of principles or to use technical methodologies. Such a way forward encounters two major problems. First, it provides no basis against which to judge the chosen priorities. Second, there is a real danger with pluralistic bargaining that there is little impetus either to use the information available, or to generate more and better information. Pluralistic bargaining presents neither real direction, nor incentives, for improving the base of knowledge and information. Future generations would therefore be in no better position for setting priorities in health care than are the policy-makers of today. These problems have been acknowledged implicitly by those setting priorities on the basis of bargaining processes, who have still chosen to use a framework against which to judge their priorities.[9,10]

Given these reservations about pursuing one approach wholeheartedly, a compromise that utilises the most advantageous aspects of each tradition, using one to inform the other, may be the best way forward. Given perfect data and perfect knowledge (both about the available alternatives and the objectives of health care), a technical priority-setting approach would be the most appropriate way forward: a technique based on the single or multiple objectives held, would be used to develop the set of priorities. In the real world, of course, there is neither perfect data nor perfect knowledge. There are, though, levels at which data and knowledge are better than at other levels. In particular, this information is better at the level of choosing alternatives within treatments and choosing alternatives within services. It may be, therefore, that these are the most appropriate levels at which to attempt to apply techniques for priority setting. At the broader level of choosing between services, data which make comparison possible are not readily available and so the level is much less appropriate for technical priority setting. At the narrowest level of choosing between patients, data that reflect the heterogeneity of patients are not available for technical priority setting. Again, the level is unlikely to be appropriate for technical priority-setting methods.

A compromise between the two approaches may therefore be to set priorities at the within-service and within-treatment levels by making the most of technical priority-setting approaches. Even at this level, however, inadequate knowledge about objectives will mean that a certain amount of pluralistic bargaining will be retained. At the broader and narrower levels, priority setting will need to rely much more heavily on opening up the political processes to debate as a way forward.

There are no empirical or theoretical examples of policies which *aim* to combine bargaining and technical approaches. Some do implicitly borrow aspects from both traditions in an attempt to make their approaches to priority setting both practical and rigorous. It has already been noted (both above and in Chapters 2 and 3) that Oregon and New Zealand have each mixed the two approaches – although in very different proportions. The efficiency-based technique of Programme Budgeting and Marginal Analysis (discussed in Chapter 5) is also heavily influenced by bargaining methods. The model of health care requirements presented later in this chapter is, however, unique in its acknowledgement, and explicit incorporation, of these two traditions.

EQUITY VERSUS EFFICIENCY

Among the technical priority-setting methodologies presented in this book, those based upon both equity and efficiency are conspicuous by their absence. In the equity models discussed in Chapter 6 it is not clear that efficiency has any impact at all. In the efficiency models discussed in Chapter 5, equity is allowed to play a part, but only as a secondary objective, once the exercise in efficiency has been completed. The technical priority-setting schemes of Oregon were based in the first instance on efficiency, and in the second on a form of equity relating to equal access for equal need (see Chapter 2). Only once the second list had been formed and the commissioners had applied their own value judgements to that list, did cost have any impact.[11] There is no doubt that cost – and thus efficiency – was an afterthought as regards this second list.

It is noticeable that in all cases *either* equity *or* efficiency provides the basis for a model, while, if it is considered at all, the other is generally tacked on at the end of the exercise in setting priorities. This may reflect the belief that only one objective is important, but it is doubtful that the tendency to restrict models to the basis of a single principle reflects either the preferences or objectives of the majority. It is much more likely that people hold both efficiency and equity objectives (although they may, of course, find these extremely difficult to express). Particularly at the extremes, where equity would be hugely compromised for the sake of efficiency, or vice versa, it is unlikely that people would be willing to pursue just one objective.

The alternative explanation is that a difficulty is experienced in incorporating more than one principle into a model for priority setting. There is little guidance from the literature about joint models, but this does not mean that it is impossible to consider both equity and efficiency in priority setting. A compromise is necessary.

How such a compromise should be effected is, however, an extremely difficult question to answer. One of the major reasons for this difficulty is that a value judgement about the importance of one objective relative to another is required. One principle must be traded off against another. People are frequently unwilling to make such value judgements explicitly. Discussion of the value basis for making such trade-offs is extremely sparse in the literature. For example, Broome discusses the need to consider both fairness and efficiency, but does not provide a resolution of the conflict.[12]

Although frameworks containing more than one principle have been developed for priority setting these have merely comprised a list of principles without statement of either the relative importance of each of the trade-offs to be made between them.[9,10] This is unsurprising. A statement of the form:

$$\text{priority} = 40\% \text{ equity} + 60\% \text{ efficiency}$$

is likely to be considered both meaningless and objectionable by many. It is informative, however, to consider explicitly how principles might be combined, even if only to conclude that this is an area that is best left to pluralistic bargaining.

For example, considering the above formula, what might the 40% refer to? One alternative might be the health care budget: 40% of the budget could be allocated on an equity basis, for example on the basis of needs assessments, and the other 60% could be allocated on the basis of efficiency, for example to maximise "health gain". There are questions, clearly, about what these numbers should be and about whether they should be constant across services/treatments. Answering these questions involves making value judgements.

An alternative means of making such trade-offs is presented in the Dutch priority-setting document *Choices in health care*.[10] This is to consider each aspect of the model in terms of the levels of support reached. In *Choices in health care* it is recommended that health care services are passed through each of four hypothetical "sieves" in turn, with each sieve representing one important aspect of health care: necessary care, effective care, efficient care and care which can be left to individual responsibility.[10] If care is deemed to be necessary, the effectiveness sieve is then to be applied. The Committee states that "Only care for which the effectiveness has been confirmed and documented belongs in the basic package" (*Choices in health care*,[10] p.86). The third sieve to be applied is that for efficiency, which will apply a lower limit to be set for inclusion in the basic package. This will be defined by low effectiveness and high cost. The final sieve to be applied retains care which it is considered can be safely left to individual responsibility. Thus, only those diagnosis/treatment combinations that fall through all four sieves will continue to form part of the basic health care package.[10]

This type of approach for the simplified example above would imply that any intervention would have to reach both a particular level of effectiveness and a particular level of cost-effectiveness before it was provided. Again, however, value judgements would be required about what these levels should be and whether they should be the same for all interventions (value judgements about which *Choices for health care* was curiously silent!). A further problem with the use of this alternative would be ensuring that levels were set such that the health care budget would be neither over – nor under – spent.

Another option has been put forward which could incorporate equity objectives more directly within an efficiency framework.[13,14] This relates to the QALY methodology. QALYs are currently formed on the basis that a QALY is equal no matter who receives it. An alternative, however, would be to weight QALYs for different types of people or different types of condition to incorporate other objectives.[13,14] Such weightings could be developed on the basis of, say, age or social class. Again, weighting in this way would involve similar types of value judgements to those discussed above.

Considering the above options is a useful exercise. It makes it quite clear that, although techniques could be developed for combining these different objectives, each is based on value judgements. At present including such explicit trade-offs in technical methodologies may be a quite unrealistic way forward. This is because of the lack of experience in making such judgements, the lack of discussion about whose place it is to make these value judgements, and the general lack of willingness to tackle such issues.

The alternative is for these judgements to be made using pluralistic bargaining methods. This avoids the need to make judgements about principles before the data concerning particular interventions are discussed by participants in the exercise. Indeed, the use now of pluralistic bargaining methods to make these judgements may provide information about values which could later be used to inform, and where appropriate be incorporated into, methodological techniques. This is the suggestion offered for the model of health care requirements advocated later in this chapter.

LAY PARTICIPATION

Chapter 7 points to the steady erosion of lay control over medicine in the UK, and Chapter 8 exposes in detail the large number of

theoretical and methodological issues surrounding public participation. The first of these chapters implies that there is little to build
from in generating a sustained debate. From the second chapter we
see the difficulty of recommending one single approach to the
incorporation of public views into pluralistic bargaining. There has
been, to date, far too little research into the theoretical and
methodological issues surrounding lay participation to recommend
any single approach. It is also true that priority setting at different
levels may require different forms of lay participation. An example
of this is provided by New Zealand's priority-setting attempts (see
Chapter 3).

New Zealand provides the main empirical example of a pluralistic
bargaining model, and goes some way towards indicating how a
framework for debate might be structured. Lay participation there
has ranged from very broad consultation and information
provision at the overall service level[15] to very specific attempts to
develop criteria based on social factors (such as the need to drive)
to define priority ratings for a variety of different illnesses.[16] There
has been little work undertaken, however, on the preferences of
individuals for different forms of participation. Although New
Zealand's experience seems to indicate that lay participation in
pluralistic bargaining can work, it does not provide any evidence
to support its choices with respect to who should be involved, at
what level, in what manner and with how much influence. What
New Zealand's experience does indicate is that the answers to
these questions are unlikely to be the same for each level of priority
setting. Abelson and colleagues have also shown, in Canada, that
preferences for involvement in different types of decision vary
considerably.[17]

The question of how much influence should be given to lay
participation is a vital one. There is still a question to be answered as
to how much the current promotion of a lay view is related to
"tokenism" on the part of the medical profession or on the part of
politicians. On the other hand, there is the worry that the aim of
incorporating a lay perspective is to absolve those in an official
capacity of their responsibility for rationing services. The elicitation
and incorporation of a lay view in health care is still very much
finding its way, and the acceptability of this basis for priority setting,

to both society at large and the patient population, is still relatively unknown.

It would certainly be dangerous to ration purely on the basis of lay preferences before further research is carried out into the probable consequences. Hence the model presented in this chapter, while recommending that public and patient preferences be incorporated, remains relatively open about how this should be achieved. The model does not prescribe the form which incorporating public preferences should take. Instead it recommends the use of different methodologies, definitions of the public, etc., in an attempt to discover the influence that these factors have on priority setting.

CONCLUSION: THE CONFUSION CLARIFIED

A great deal of confusion has surrounded the area of priority setting in health care. This has come about, at least in part, because of the broad basis of contribution to the debate by those of diverse disciplinary traditions with differing terminology and inadequate understanding of other branches of learning. Sadly, the different disciplinary traditions have generally been unable either to communicate or to work together in order to further the development of adequate policy. Frequently the discussion of priority setting by academics has become divorced from the practice of priority setting at all levels. Nothing shows this more clearly than the work of Klein and colleagues on the lack of practical progress shown by health authorities in this area.[18]

Various options for priority setting are outlined throughout this book. The technical options, though, are hindered both by their ambition and their narrow ethical basis. Pluralistic bargaining is limited by the, as yet unanswered, question of how to incorporate a lay viewpoint and how to ensure that such bargaining is based on the best available information. There are thus disadvantages in pursuing each of these routes in isolation from the other. The next section of this chapter presents and discusses the model of health care requirements: a potential way forward for priority setting.

ACCEPTING THE CONFLICT: A WAY FORWARD

In this final section of the final chapter of this book, a means of carrying the priority-setting debate forward is proposed. This is the model of health care requirements, the main characteristics of which are shown in Table 9.1. This version is substantially altered from that previously reported in Ref. 20. The model of health care requirements draws upon the strengths of both technical priority setting and pluralistic bargaining. Technical priority setting is based on the pursuit of explicit objectives: in this model equity and efficiency principles are combined to provide a framework for priority setting. Pluralistic bargaining acknowledges the need to set priorities at different levels and this notion, too, is incorporated into the model – as is the need to incorporate a lay viewpoint. The model also, however, accepts and works within the conflicts that arise. Although equity and efficiency are explicitly incorporated into the model they are traded off using consensus methods rather than specific techniques. Although lay participation is strongly advocated,

Table 9.1 Summary of the characteristics of the health care requirements approach to priority setting

Health Care Requirements
• Aims to provide a framework for priority setting now, but by combining this with the research agenda, to inform methods for priority setting in the future.
• Combines the advantages of pluralistic bargaining with those of technical priority setting.
• Incorporates principles of equity (based on need) and efficiency.
• Pluralistic bargaining, within the framework proposed by health care requirements, provides a basis for priority setting at most levels.
• Pluralistic bargaining incorporates a lay viewpoint – but is not prescriptive about the form this should take.
• Technical priority setting is directed at particular areas where there appears to be potential for change.
• Technical priority setting is based on three steps for action: consensus, literature review, dedicated research.
• Within technical priority setting, trade-offs between principles are based on bargaining approaches.

the model is deliberately not prescriptive about the form that lay participation should take because of the debate surrounding how best to incorporate a lay viewpoint.

THE GENERAL STRUCTURE OF THE MODEL

Incorporating a Research Agenda

Any way forward in the priority-setting debate must combine a means of setting priorities now, with the potential for improving the ability to set priorities in the future. It is not sufficient, then, to find a means of setting priorities that is comfortable at the current time. Means of priority setting in the future can be informed by incorporating research alongside the current attempts to set priorities. One of the major advantages of using pluralistic bargaining in conjunction with technical priority setting is that it can facilitate this process. For example, the trade-offs between equity and efficiency that are made in practice using pluralistic bargaining, may inform more precise means of making these trade-offs in the future. Similarly the difficult issues surrounding the acquisition of public preferences (as discussed in Chapter 8) will in large part be informed by analytical assessment of practical attempts to include a lay viewpoint in current priority-setting exercises. The model of health care requirements therefore calls for the inclusion of the research alongside the current attempts to set priorities.

Three Essential Principles

The model of health care requirements is based on three essential principles for priority setting. The first of these principles is based on equity, the second on efficiency and the third principle is that of lay participation – and particularly, patient acceptability. The equity principle advocates equal treatment on the basis of equal need, where the definition of need is that the patient should have the capacity to benefit from treatment. Thus, there should be equal treatment of patients who have equal ability to benefit from care. The efficiency principle is based on the notion of maximising (rather than equalising) ability to benefit in terms of improved health. Choices between different types of care (for this principle) are based on their relative cost–utility. The practical expression of efficiency is cost–utility analysis because its objective – to maximise health-related utility – is assumed to be closer to the objective of the health care system than the objectives of cost–benefit analysis. The final principle, that of lay participation, and particularly patient preferences, is treated differently at each of the different levels of priority setting.

Priority Setting at Different Levels

Priority setting must be considered differently at different levels. Although there are a number of levels at which priority setting can be considered, the model of health care requirements defines four such levels.

1. Priority setting across whole services – comparisons which might be made would be, for example, mental health versus child health, or community care versus acute hospital care, or elective surgery versus life-threatening illness.
2. Priority setting within services, but across treatments – an example might be setting priorities between hip replacement and arthroscopy in orthopaedic surgery.
3. Priority setting within treatments – an example might be, for prostatectomy, setting priorities between those with chronic urinary retention and those with severe urinary symptoms.
4. Priority setting between individual patients. At this level priority setting will involve taking into account the individual characteristics of patients and their own preferences.

At each of these different levels there will need to be different mixes of the technical and bargaining traditions of priority setting. It is certainly not expected within the model of health care requirements that detailed technical analysis should be applied to all aspects of health care. Indeed this would be impractical given the complexities and costs of research in health care, and the practical difficulties of obtaining valid and reliable results. Technical priority setting – or detailed analysis – should therefore be incorporated into selected areas, within a system more generally based on pluralistic bargaining. Conversely, pluralistic bargaining – with the health care requirements framework as a background – can be used to inform those levels of priority setting where technical methods would currently be inappropriate.

At the level of priority setting across whole services, there is insufficient information for technical methods to provide anything at all meaningful. At this level, therefore, pluralistic bargaining should inform the different decisions that must be made. This bargaining will be informed by a variety of general debates such as the treatment of the young versus that of the old, the treatment of so-called self-inflicted conditions versus the treatment of "victims" of disease, as well as general considerations of effectiveness and cost-effectiveness.

Pluralistic bargaining, as well as providing the main basis for priority setting at the very broadest levels, must also be the primary focus at the most detailed level: at the level of setting priorities between patients. Here, technical solutions are unlikely to cope adequately with the heterogeneity of patients. They will be unable to provide the flexibility required when patients differ widely and have many differing variants of the same conditions. At this level, it is for the clinician, in conjunction with the preferences of the patient, to set priorities: joint decision-making by clinicians and patients[19,21] using open and explicit methods could thus contribute to allocation decisions between patients.

For priority setting within conditions and across conditions the use of technical analyses may be more feasible. Thus, at this level, the technical schema of health care requirements may be applied.

THE TECHNICAL SCHEMA

The technical aspect of the health care requirements model involves explicitly assessing information about each of the three essential principles upon which priorities are to be based. The equity principle should be based upon the examination of the distribution of remediable disease within the population (equity of access according to ability to benefit) – and therefore is reliant upon information about effectiveness as well as prevalence and incidence. Efficiency should be taken into account by combining information on costs with information on effectiveness (in the form of utility). Public and patient preferences are also incorporated into the detailed schema: of particular importance within this schema is information about whether or not proposed treatments are acceptable to the patient group(s) under consideration.

Grand plans and statements of intent are associated with most techniques that are advocated for the purposes of priority setting, and generally these models are unsuccessful in achieving their objectives. It is important here, therefore, to stress three particular aspects of this technical schema within the health care requirements model. First, it is not intended that all the possible areas of health care intervention should be investigated using technical methodologies at one time. Second, the scheme contains three practical steps for action. Third, even this technical element of the model contains aspects of pluralistic bargaining. Each of these aspects will be discussed in turn.

Choice of Intervention

In practice it will take much time and hard work before the health service is able to set priorities using technical methodologies – even in the limited areas of setting priorities within conditions and within specialties/services. This is recognised here and therefore detailed consideration of selected areas, within the general framework of debate and rational choice, is advocated. Fitting particular areas into the general framework will be difficult and is likely to take place on a relatively crude basis, but it is, in any case, impractical to attempt to change the whole pattern of services at one time. The process could be seen as analogous to doing a jigsaw in which certain parts of the picture are concentrated on at any one time.

Particular areas of health care may be chosen for more detailed study on a number of bases. Areas of concern may include interventions aimed at treating particular common and expensive conditions, for example stroke; interventions which aim to service particular client groups, for example the mental health services; interventions which have something particular in common, for example the large-volume elective surgery conditions; interventions from one particular specialty; etc. It is important, however, that the not inconsiderable resources involved in applying the detailed schema of health care requirements, should be allocated, at least in the first instance, to areas of particular uncertainty or confusion or where current priorities seem to be manifestly at odds with those suggested by the (limited) information available. The areas with the greatest potential for change would appear to be the most important areas on which to focus.

Three Steps for Action

Having chosen a specific aspect of health care intervention for study, three steps for action are advocated, as shown below. Each step should consider carefully the evidence for the three essential aspects of priority setting: the population distribution of remediable disease (combining information on effectiveness with information about distribution), cost-effectiveness, and public and patient preference which, as outlined above, enable the process of priority setting to take into account the principles of equity and efficiency, and which allow the incorporation of a lay viewpoint.

1. Developing priorities on the basis of easily accessible information.
2. Developing priorities on the basis of detailed examination of existing literature and routinely available data.
3. Developing priorities on the basis of dedicated research to discover the population distribution, effectiveness, cost-effectiveness, and public preferences, for the chosen health care interventions.

Step 1

The first step in the detailed schema of health care requirements is to provide a basis for priority setting by obtaining consensus based on easily accessible information – including the experience of clinicians. In particular, priority setting at this level may involve the use of consensus conferences. Such consensus might usually be obtained from experts in the field, but it is recommended that those involved in making these decisions should include other parties. Lay viewpoints might well be provided by patients suffering from particular illnesses, representatives from groups with a special interest in a disease or service, or general patient advocates such as members of the Community Health Councils. In many ways, apart from the health care requirements framework which provides a basis for the information which should be considered in obtaining consensus, this first level differs very little from what might be expected in a pure pluralistic bargaining approach and is very similar to much of the work conducted in New Zealand. At this level, the method also has similarities with programme budgeting and marginal analysis as advocated by Mooney et al.[22] For the purposes of the health care requirements model, however, the analysis should consider each of the three essential aspects of priority setting, and should not be limited exclusively to the consideration of efficiency. The areas within which priorities are to be set are also chosen on a more technical basis in this health care requirements schema (for example, areas where medical practice variation is high, thus indicating a greater extent of confusion) than in the programme budgeting approach, where areas of interest are defined by the bargaining group.

Step 2

The second step within the health care requirements model is to consider systematically the existing literature and routinely available data. This is not a small task – hence it forms the second step in defining health care requirements rather than the first! It is important that these analyses consider the evidence regarding the population distribution of indications for an intervention, the effectiveness of treatment, the cost-effectiveness of treatment and any information on the public or patients' desire for the intervention to be provided. Such forms of analysis are becoming increasingly common internationally, and are supported in the UK by the Department of Health who have funded the production of both the Effective Health Care Bulletins[23] and the Epidemiologically Based Needs Assessments.[24,25] The development of the Cochrane Collaboration and methodologies for systematic review also provide assistance for those interpreting the literature.[26] In themselves, these analyses are useful for considering priorities within the treatment of particular conditions, and can contribute information for setting priorities within services when combined with other similar analyses. Each review alone, however, is of course insufficient for the purpose of priority setting across condtions, in that it is unlikely to involve comparisons between different conditions, and does not always set the particular intervention in the context even of its own specialty.

Step 3

The third step is to perform dedicated research in each of the three essential areas. Research should concentrate on those aspects not informed by the detailed literature reviews. This research should include assessment of each of the three essential attributes of priority setting, and the methodology used should enable the maximisation of the research potential from limited resources. One potential methodology would be to assess the population distribution of remediable disease by conducting studies of the prevalence and incidence of the chosen conditions in specific areas. This would then be combined with assessment of the effectiveness (or outcome) of intervention. Similarly information about the cost-effectiveness of treatment must be obtained. Both effectiveness and cost data may potentially be obtained via observational studies, with untreated patients being identified from studies of the population, or where possible in experimental studies. The public desire for the treatment of particular conditions will need to be assessed using both qualitative and quantitative methods, but the form which the incorporation of a lay viewpoint should take is left relatively open in this schema. It is of vital importance that a patient perspective on the acceptability of the treatment is included, but it will also be appropriate to incorporate other lay views. Given the difficulties in acquiring a lay view – or even in determining what is meant by a lay view – it is impossible to be overly prescriptive at present about how this should be done. Instead, it is recommended that a variety of means of incorporating a lay viewpoint are experimented with, thus enabling more informed attempts in the future.

The Contribution of Each Step to Priority Setting

It is important to consider how each of these steps can contribute to the overall priority-setting process. The first step is intended to provide a short-term solution, particularly for those interventions where there is likely to be insufficient evidence contained in the existing literature. While such consensus of opinion is unlikely to be adequate in the longer term, it can give purchasers some basis for priority setting where the existing information is inadequate. The second step provides a medium-term solution. Literature review and routine data analysis could potentially provide information about each of the three areas of interest. It is likely, however, that in many cases the research will be either inadequate or non-existent.[27-32] In the medium term, however, consensus based on the material contained in such reviews will provide purchasing authorities with at least some basis for the decisions that they must take. Where reviews show that there is already adequate information for the setting of priorities this information can be used and the final step need not be pursued. It is when the evidence upon which decisions are reached is inadequate that the third step is required. The carrying out of rigorous research in this step will provide detailed information for the setting of priorities in the long term and must then be combined with empirically obtained data about public preferences.

Pluralistic Bargaining and the "Balance Sheet" Approach

Because each of the different principles is considered explicitly within the technical schema, the resulting priorities are less likely to suffer from omissions of important data than many of the other bases for priority setting described earlier in the book. Introduced, however, is the problem of trading one principle against another. In the first section of this chapter, consideration was given to the problems associated with trading off the different principles which inform the priority-setting process. Three means of trading off one principle against another were mentioned, none of which seems to be a practical way of taking these value judgements forward at this time.

It is therefore assumed that within the schema of health care requirements this trading-off of one principle against another will be initially accomplished by bargaining processes. These bargaining processes may, in turn, inform more precise value judgements about these trade-offs. It is advocated here that a "balance sheet" approach be used to assist in this decision-making. These "balance sheets" should contain all the available information regarding the principles outlined above for each of the interventions being considered. Ideally this information should be collected for differing severities of each condition. An example of such a balance sheet is shown in Table 9.2, which utilises data on hips and knees obtained from the Epidemiologically Based Needs Assessments. The information found through these literature reviews was insufficient to be able to classify those requiring hip or knee replacement, on the basis of severity of condition. It is quite apparent that attempts to form such balance sheets at the present time suffer from the poor quality of much available data, and thus it is essential that information about data quality should comprise part of the balance sheet. Schemas for the assessment of the quality of evidence thus need to be devised which can be applied to each area. These will need to be similar to the proforma developed to assess quality of effectiveness evidence by the US Preventive Services Task Force,[33] and adapted by Williams et al.[30] This is used to assess the quality of the evidence on effectiveness in Table 9.2. It is vital that, where evidence is relatively poor (for example regarding the comparative cost-effectiveness of the different procedures), this is acknowledged.

On the basis of the information contained in such balance sheets, those involved in taking the decisions can decide which specific treatments for which specific severities of illness should be considered priorities. These decisions will involve making value judgements about the relative importance of each of the different principles, as well as assessing the information available for the specific conditions. Although the use of bargaining in this way may not be considered sufficiently scientific or technical by some, it is impossible to recommend an alternative unless those setting priorities are willing to commit themselves to a predetermined basis for trading off one principle against another. Even if health care purchasers are willing to make such defined trade-offs, they may be hindered in practice by information that varies in quality across the different principles.

It may be argued that many health authorities already implicitly combine this sort of information. It is important, however, that each

Table 9.2 An example of the balance sheet approach comparing the treatments of hip replacement and knee replacement

	Population distribution of need for surgery	Q	Effectiveness	Q	Cost-effectiveness	Q	Public preferences	Q
Knees – treatment by total knee replacement (TKR)	0.03% aged 45–54, 0.03% aged 55–64, 0.17% aged 65–74, 0.18% aged 75+[27]		Pain relief and satisfactory function in 90% cases, but deep wound infection occurs in 0.5–2% cases, and for all cases there is a 2–3% probability of revision after 6 years[27]	III	Estimates of cost per QALY for TKR vary considerably from £1600 to £7810 for knee OA		None	
Hips – treatment by total hip replacement	1.2% aged 65+[36]		72–100% obtain pain relief and improved mobility, but 5–10% of patients experience complications. There is a 1–2% failure rate per annum[28]	III	Three estimates of cost per QALY are available: £750 (1983 price),[33] £699 and £330[34]		None	

Based on Refs 29 and 32. Q = quality of evidence (based on levels from I (best) to IV (poorest)); III indicates "Opinions of respected authorities, based on clinical experience, descriptive studies or reports of expert committees".[32]

of the different forms of data is explicitly considered and compared across the interventions for which the decision is being made. Detailed and methodical scrutiny of each of the component areas is required before any decision is made. It is important to stress here that this model does not require that any principle be subordinate to any other: in some cases public preferences may be felt to override effectiveness, for example, but in other cases the opposite may be true.

Pluralistic bargaining forms a major part of the schema of health care requirements, although at each of the distinct steps there are different emphases on the extent to which bargaining is involved in the priority-setting process. Within the first step the emphasis is very much on the bargaining process. Although a framework is provided, it is expected that those involved in developing consensus will bring their own objectives to the bargaining table. In the second step, the emphasis on the information contained in the balance sheet is much greater, although consensus will still be required both where information is poor and for the trading-off aspect of setting the priorities. In the third step the information provided should be good, and the main aspect of bargaining will be in trading off the different principles. At all three levels of priority setting within the health care requirements schema, therefore, decisions must be made in terms of the extent to which one principle is traded against another.

LAY PARTICIPATION AND HEALTH CARE REQUIREMENTS

Who is involved in decision-making may be of vital importance in the results that are obtained throughout the model of health care requirements – not just at the levels which incorporate technical priority methods. It is recommended here that lay input should always be included in this decision-making body. The form that this lay input should take is, however, questionable. It could be that a lay viewpoint could come from "experts" of some sort, such as patients or their representatives. Alternatively it could come from elected or appointed officials, or it could come from the interested citizenry. It is important to indicate, however, that further research is required to determine the most useful and effective methods to allow public participation within the health care requirements model. Indeed, in different locations, different lay representatives may be considered more or less appropriate for this role. One option would be to set up an advisory group with whom the bargaining questions (at each of the top three levels) could be tackled. Such a group could then provide advice to those responsible for setting priorities.

The only area in which the health care requirements model is prescriptive with regard to lay participation is at the level of setting priorities between patients, where a patient should be involved in the decisions about the treatment that they should receive. A view about the acceptability of procedures to particular patient groups should also be included within the technical schema at the levels of priority setting between and within treatments for different conditions.

A prerequisite for pluralistic bargaining is, of course, an atmosphere of debate which will inform decision-making. A wide range of issues will need to be discussed, particularly concerning who will be involved in decision-making and how their preferences will be combined. Lessons about how to generate such debate could be learned from those priority-setting exercises that have already been conducted, such as those in New Zealand and Oregon. Chapter 8 contains methods for obtaining information about people's views that could also be useful in engendering discussion.

IMPLEMENTING THE MODEL OF HEALTH CARE REQUIREMENTS

The schema of health care requirements can be used to define priorities. At each level, judgement will be used to decide, on the basis of the balance sheet and the available budget, which specific treatments for which specific severities of illness should be considered priorities. Essentially this will result in a decision, albeit a relatively crude and approximate decision, on the proportion of funding to be allocated to different alternatives. Once this decision has been made, however, the question of implementing the chosen priorities becomes important. This could be done through providing a budget for a particular condition and allowing clinicians to distribute it among patients with that condition in the way they choose; or more prescriptively, by producing guidelines for treatments of specific severities of illness (which may, of course, include exclusions for certain types of patients in usual circumstances); or it may even include directives about which patients to treat in all circumstances. The latter is the most unlikely option given the heterogeneity of patients, and would almost certainly have to be combined with a good appeals procedure for patients with "unusual" circumstances.

Whichever option is chosen, it is inevitable that there will be attempts at times to bypass the priorities, hence the concern voiced in the first section of this chapter that other incentives to follow priorities must also be developed.

CONCLUSION

This chapter has established the foundation for an approach to priority setting which is unique in that it acknowledges the need to incorporate both technical methodologies and bargaining techniques. In practice all methods draw from both traditions (as shown in the empirical examples of Oregon and New Zealand discussed in Chapters 2 and 3) but there has been little acknowledgement of this reality. Instead the various disciplines have been content to promote their own alternatives, taking little note of the advances being made elsewhere. The multidisciplinary approach to priority setting advocated here has aimed to set aside the confusion generated, accept the complexity of the problem, and acknowledge the contributions that can be made by a range of traditions.

The model of health care requirements is only one approach to priority setting; of course there are others. The health care requirements framework provides a practical method for setting priorities based on existing data. Further, with its concurrent research agenda, there is the opportunity for future development. While the essential principles included in the description above are set in the context of the UK in the mid-1990s, the flexibility of the model would allow different objectives to be appropriately represented on the balance sheet at other times and in other societies.

Index

Index compiled by Jill Halliday